Pain from

Unrelated Treatment

Mission Statement

IASP brings together scientists, clinicians, healthcare providers, and policy makers to stimulate and support the study of pain and to translate that knowledge into improved pain relief worldwide. IASP Press publishes timely, high-quality, and reasonably priced books relating to pain research and treatment.

Pain from Unrelated Treatment

Editor:

John Jarrell, MD, MSc, FRCSC
Professor
Department of Obstetrics and Gynecology
Cumming School of Medicine
University of Calgary
Department of Obstetrics and Gynecology
Foothills Medical Center
Calgary, Alberta,
Canada
And
Calgary Chronic Pain Centre
Alberta Health Services,
Calgary, Alberta,
Canada

International Association for the Study of Pain
IASP®
Working together for pain relief

Wolters Kluwer
Philadelphia • Baltimore • New York • London
Buenos Aires • Hong Kong • Sydney • Tokyo

Acquisitions Editor: Keith Donnellan
Development Editor: Sean McGuire
Production Project Manager: Barton Dudlick
Design Coordinator: Joan Wendt
Manufacturing Coordinator: Beth Welsh
Marketing Manager: Stacy Malyil
Prepress Vendor: Aptara, Inc.

ISBN: 9781975103064

Published by:
IASP Press®
International Association for the Study of Pain
111 Queen Anne Ave N, Suite 501
Seattle, WA 98109-4955, USA
Fax: 206-283-9403
www.iasp-pain.org

Printed in China

Library of Congress Cataloging-in-Publication Data

Names: Jarrell, John F., editor. | International Association for the Study of Pain, issuing body.
Title: Pain from unrelated treatment / editor, John Jarrell.
Description: Philadelphia : Wolters Kluwer Health, Lippincott Williams & Wilkins, [2019]
Identifiers: LCCN 2018025171 | ISBN 9781975103064
Subjects: | MESH: Pain, Postoperative | Pain, Procedural | Surgical Procedures, Operative–adverse effects | Therapeutics–adverse effects
Classification: LCC RB127 | NLM WO 184 | DDC 616/.0472–dc23
LC record available at https://lccn.loc.gov/2018025171

LWW.com

CCS0618

CONTRIBUTORS

Asbjørn Mohr Drewes, MD, PhD, DMSc, EDPM
Professor (Chair) and Chief Physician
Director of Mech-Sense and Centre for Pancreatic Diseases
Department of Gastroenterology and Hepatology
Clinical Institute at Aalborg University Hospital
Aalborg, Denmark

Steven R. Hanling, MD
Department of Anesthesiology
Medical College of Georgia
Augusta University
Augusta, Georgia

Joseph E. LaGrew II, MD
Department of Anesthesiology
College of Medicine
University of Florida
Gainesville, Florida

Rajiv Midha, MD, MSc
Professor and Department Head
Department of Clinical Neurosciences
Hotchkiss Brain Institute
University of Calgary
Department Head
Department of Clinical Neurosciences
Foothills Medical Center
Calgary, Alberta

Sudheesh Ramachandran, MCh
Clinical Fellow (Peripheral Nerve Surgery)
Department of Clinical Neurosciences
Hotchkiss Brain Institute
University of Calgary
Clinical Fellow
Department of Clinical Neurosciences
Foothills Medical Center
Calgary, Alberta

Magali Robert, MD, MSc
Professor
Department of Obstetrics and Gynecology
Cumming School of Medicine
University of Calgary
Division of Pelvic Medicine and Reconstructive Surgery
Department of Obstetrics and Gynecology
Foothills Medical Center
Calgary, Alberta

Carter H. Sigmon, MD
Department of Anesthesiology
Naval Medical Center San Diego
San Diego, California

Karen Walker-Bone, BM, FRCP, PhD
Professor of Occupational Rheumatology
MRC Lifecourse Epidemiology Unit
University of Southampton
Honorary Consultant in Rheumatology
Southampton General Hospital
Southampton, United Kingdom

PREFACE

The purpose of this book is to describe the experience of pain that can occur in a number of frequently utilized medical treatments and procedures. The conditions discussed in this book are quite disparate in nature. They represent treatments and procedures for painful and nonpainful conditions with high rates of utilization. The focus of each chapter is pain as a consequence of previous treatment. While the treatments are diverse, so too are the pain mechanisms and experiences. In some cases such as the administration of statins and the insertion of pelvic mesh, the treatments have been controversial.

The consideration of pain in some cases such as abdominal and pelvic surgery has been challenging, as the indication of the underlying disease is pre-existing pain itself. The complete assessment has required appreciation of the possibility of a new pain mechanism versus the continuation of the pretreatment pain state. The subjects under review required a broad understanding of the physiology of each system under review, the impact of disease itself on pain, as well as the separation in some instances of a new posttreatment pain mechanism and proposed treatment.

Overall the book outlines a diversity of therapies and an exploration of complex pain mechanisms. Treatments include the medical management of HIV and elevated cholesterol. Procedural treatments include dural puncture, abdominal surgery, gynecologic laparoscopy, as well as the insertion of pelvic mesh as a treatment for pelvic relaxation.

Dr. Karen Walker-Bone has provided an extensive summary of HIV, its association with pain, and the pain resulting from treatment with antiretroviral therapy. The risks of chronic pain are explored associated with the disease that relate to the viral load. Pain management is discussed and recognized as underutilized at present, presenting an added challenge to this complex disease.

Drs. Sudheesh Ramachandran and Rajiv Midha have reviewed our current understanding of nerve injury. The authors provide a detailed exploration of the mechanisms of neuropathic pain as well as other iatrogenic nerve injuries. Treatment options are explored fully while recommending caution in relation to further surgery in most instances.

Drs. Joseph E. LaGrew, Carter H. Sigmon, and Steven R. Hanling have explored the common problem of postdural puncture headache. Historically, postdural headache emerged from self-experimentation with cocaine. The potential mechanisms of pain are described as well as the important differential diagnosis in the postpartum state. Basic and modifiable risks and mitigating approaches are described as well as active treatment approaches.

Dr. Asbjørn Mohr Drewes has described the pathophysiology of painful gastrointestinal visceral disease and the pain resulting from procedures to eliminate painful conditions. Preventative approaches are presented among those at risk of chronicity. Active treatment approaches are discussed.

Dr. John Jarrell has explored a similar consideration of painful visceral disease of the pelvis that is commonly complicated by the emergence of a chronic pain state following treatment. Overinterpretation of pain from small areas of endometriosis as a result of misattribution bias can result in less active treatment of dysmenorrhea, a very common cause of chronic pelvic pain. Active pain testing at the bedside is encouraged to gain a more fulsome understanding of the woman's pain experience.

Dr. Magali Robert has explored the controversial application of mesh into the pelvis for the management of pelvic floor prolapse. Variances in stakeholder reports of success prompt a recommendation for better assessment of patient pain status before implementation of treatments like artificial mesh insertion and the comparison to native tissues to gain clearer appreciation of possible benefit.

Dr. John Jarrell has reviewed current understanding related to the commonly administered statin medication for the prevention of cardiovascular disease. This treatment has resulted in the emergence of a pain state that ranges from mild discomfort to a rarely experienced lethal outcome. The biochemical mechanisms of pain are explored. International reports that are directed to the management of pain are presented.

It has been a privilege to participate in this project with such knowledgeable and capable clinicians and scientists. I want to express my appreciation for their participation and in some cases completion of tasks despite major personal challenges.

John Jarrell

It has been a pleasure to participate as an editor in this project as the authors have completed their commitments despite in some cases significant personal challenges.

CONTENTS

CHAPTER 1

Pain Associated with HIV and Antiretroviral Therapy

Karen Walker-Bone

HIV is a global pandemic. According to the World Health Organization, there are an estimated 37 million people worldwide living with HIV, with >3 million of those children aged <15 years.[51] The vast majority (an estimated 24.7 million) of people living with HIV (PLWHIV) are in sub-Saharan Africa; around 5 million in Asia and the Pacific region; more than 2.3 million in North America, Western, and Central Europe; and 1.6 million in Latin America.[51] Untreated, people can live with asymptomatic infection for a variable duration but ultimately the virus is associated with severe immunodeficiency leading to opportunistic infections and malignancies and premature death. In one of the most dramatic and rapid phases of drug development ever seen and as a result of a hitherto unseen levels of cooperation between pharmaceutical companies and worldwide regulatory authorities, the first antiretroviral therapy (ART) became available in the 1990s. Over the subsequent years, there have been substantial advances in the treatment of HIV infection, and in developed countries where access to treatment is widely available life expectancy approaches normal.[33] This has led to a growing population of people with chronic prevalent, treated infection living to older ages. This chapter will provide an overview of what is known about pain among PLWHIV, considering risk factors, impact, sites of pain, and adequacy of treatment. It should however be borne in mind that most of the research into PLWHIV has taken place in the resource-rich nations and may not generalize to the entire global population.

PREVALENCE AND INCIDENCE OF PAIN IN HIV

The earliest data about pain and HIV came from studies among patients with advanced infection or AIDS[4,6,41] often in palliative care settings.[25,48] In these patients, pain was a very common symptom.[4,44,30] For example, in one of the most important early studies, Breitbart et al. surveyed 438 ambulatory AIDS patients and found that 60% of subjects reported pain with an average pain intensity of 5.4/10 and significant functional impairment.[6] In their prospective longitudinal study, Frich and Borgbjerg[16] reported a prevalence of pain of 74% at baseline and an incidence of pain of 88% among 95 AIDS patients over 2 years of follow-up.

Parker et al.[42] published a systematic review of the studies of the prevalence of pain in PLWHIV in 2015. Including 28 papers published over 18 years through the pre-ART and post-ART era (1993–2011), they estimated a point prevalence of pain of 54% (95% CI 51.14–56.09), a 3-month period estimate of 83% (95% CI 76–88), and a 6-month period estimate of 72% (95% CI 68.7–76.3). Notably, most of the research on pain had been conducted in the United States, Canada, and Europe but they were able to include studies from South Africa ($n = 5$), Brazil ($n = 1$), India ($n = 1$), Vietnam ($n = 1$), and Nigeria ($n = 1$). They noted remarkably little change in the estimated rates of pain across all the studies even despite the changing nature and availability of ART.[42]

Wilson et al.[56] reported on the symptom burden of a cohort of PLWHIV, all of whom had access to ART. The most prevalent and bothersome symptoms were muscle aches/joint pain, fatigue, and poor sleep. The results of this study suggest that, even with the most modern, improved ART regimens, pain remains a common and troublesome symptom, associated with a high level of distress. Similar findings have been reported recently in France[5] and Australia.[10]

SITES OF PAIN IN HIV

Many of the early studies did not classify pain by anatomical site or focused only on specific sites or types of pain, such as pleuritic[29] or neuropathic pain.[53] In their study among ambulatory HIV-positive patients, Singer et al.[49] described a point prevalence of pain of 28% among asymptomatic HIV-positive patients and 80% among AIDS patients ($p = 0.001$) with back and joint pain the two most common sites affected. In Canada, McCormack et al.[34] found that 55% of 148 ambulatory HIV patients had experienced HIV-associated pain in the preceding month, with the most common sites: legs (43%), back (38%), head (31%), arms/hands (29%), anogenital/pelvic (28%), and abdomen (27%). Similarly, in an investigation of 104 AIDS patients (63% women, 4% on ARVs) in South Africa, 98% of subjects reported pain with 66% reporting the lower limbs as the most prevalent site.[41] Among a case-control study of 61 HIV-infected children as compared with 61 noninfected controls, infected children were five-fold more likely to report pain (OR 5.3, 95% CI 2–14.3) than those without and the most common sites were the abdomen, lower limbs, and headache.[30] Rotheram-Borus et al. found that 83% of 151 patients with advanced AIDS reported experiencing physical pain, 75% of whom reported joint/muscle pain.[47] Martin et al.[32] also found that the intravenous drug users reported pain at a higher mean number of sites (2.4 vs. 1.9, $p < 0.05$) again with the most marked effect in the group classified as asymptomatic.

In their systematic review, Parker et al.[42] found that 14/28 included studies reported on the number of anatomical sites affected. The number of sites ranged from a median of 1 (1–2) found in the rural South African study to a median of 2.5 (1–5) in the New York study.[6] Studies varied in the distribution and number of sites of pain that were asked about making them difficult to pool but all 28 studies included the lower limbs, which were the most commonly affected site, with headache or head/neck pain the next most common. In 2011, Kamerman and Mitchell[24] published a review of the pain studies in sub-Saharan Africa and did not find any differences in the number or distribution of sites described in the African studies as compared with the studies from resource-rich

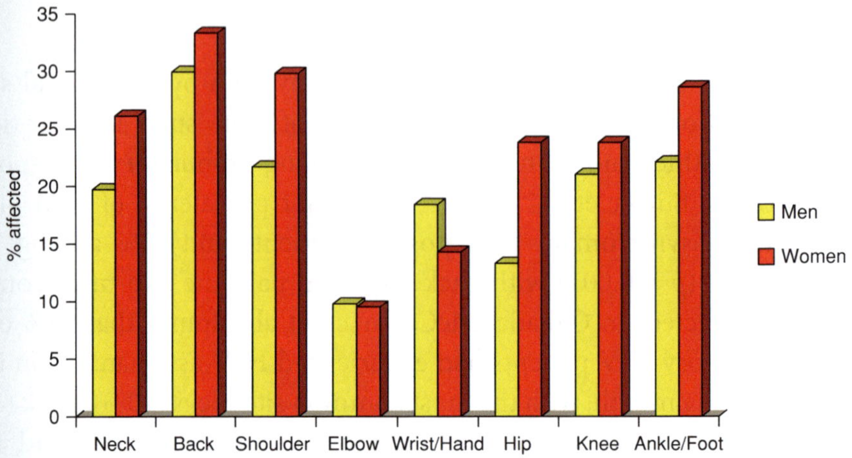

FIGURE 1-1 Prevalence of pain lasting at least 1 week over the past 1 month by regional site in 859 PLWHIV. (Data from Lawson E, Sabin C, Perry N, et al. Is HIV painful? An epidemiologic study of the prevalence and risk factors for pain in HIV-infected patients. *Clin J Pain*. 2015;31:813–819.)

countries. In comparison, data from a UK cohort study (Fig. 1-1) showed that back pain was the most common single site affected. However, pooling pain data from hips, knees, and ankle/feet would similarly make lower limb pain the most common.[28] In this chapter, the authors noted an excess of pain in the foot/ankle among PLWHIV as compared with the general population pain studies.

RISK FACTORS FOR PAIN

Risk factors for pain have been evaluated in a number of different studies but few investigators were comprehensive in their consideration of relevant factors and it must be borne in mind that most of the studies did not include an HIV-negative control group.

Demographic Factors

We found few studies in which age has been treated as an independent risk factor for pain. However, in a UK cross-sectional study including >850 PLWHIV, age was an independent statistically significant risk

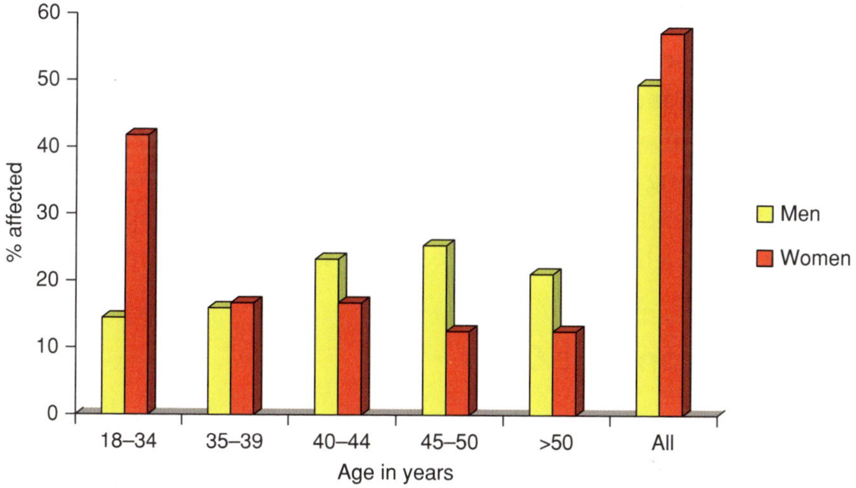

FIGURE 1-2 Prevalence of chronic pain (lasting at least 3 months) by age and gender among 859 PLWHIV. (Data from Lawson E, Sabin C, Perry N, et al. Is HIV painful? An epidemiologic study of the prevalence and risk factors for pain in HIV-infected patients. *Clin J Pain*. 2015;31:813–819.)

factor for pain lasting more than 1 day in the past month ($p < 0.001$) and for chronic pain (lasting more than 3 months) ($p = 0.004$).[28] In some, but not all, studies HIV-positive women have been found significantly more likely to report pain than men.[3,6,28,41] Moreover, in some studies women also reported pain of a more severe intensity than men.[6,28] In their systematic review, Parker et al.[42] found that 6 of the 28 included studies reported on demographic factors and pain. Of these, 2/6 reported a higher rate of prevalence of pain among women as compared with men[6,39] but one study in South Africa found the converse.[20] In a UK study comparing the prevalence of chronic pain (lasting at least 3 months) by age and gender, women reported pain more commonly than men overall, but the most marked differences were found among the youngest women surveyed (aged 18 to 34 years) in whom the rate of prevalence was 41% among women as compared with 14% among men (Fig. 1-2). Women in pain were also significantly more likely than men in pain to report that they were taking analgesics most days for their pain ($p < 0.0001$).[28]

As far as ethnicity is concerned, the data are inconclusive: Richardson et al. included US women from Caucasian, African American, and

Hispanic backgrounds and showed no differences in pain severity or frequency among women of different ethnicities,[33] but Rotheram-Borus[47] found ethnic variations such that subjects of Latino origin expressed more pain symptoms and pain distress than African Americans. Among the studies included in the Parker systematic review, two studies found a higher prevalence of pain in black respondents[2,13] and one found a higher prevalence in non-Caucasian groups.[6]

Socioeconomic Class

Lower socioeconomic class has been found associated with an increased prevalence of pain in some studies.[38,39]

Educational Attainment

Although rarely included as a risk factor, two studies found a higher prevalence of pain among those with lower levels of educational attainment.[13,39]

Lifestyle Factors

Alcohol and illicit drug use are prevalent among PLWHIV. Richardson et al.[46] found that cigarette smoking was associated with pain severity (current smoking OR 2.22, 95% CI 1.36–3.63) and frequency (current smoking OR 1.79, 95% CI 1.1–2.91). Interestingly, exploring the factors associated with effective abstinence from cigarette smoking, Aigner et al.[1] recently showed that lower levels of pain at baseline were associated with increased likelihood of successful smoking cessation treatment, no matter how the cessation treatment was delivered. There has not been any consistent positive or negative association between pain and alcohol in HIV.[46]

A number of researchers have explored the relationship between illicit drug use and pain.[6,11,13,18,32,46] Almost all studies found a significantly increased prevalence and intensity of pain among those with a history of intravenous drug use (IVDU), as compared with those without.[11,13,18,32,46] In contrast, Breitbart et al.[6] found no differences by IVDU. In one study, Marijuana or hash use was significantly associated with severity of pain (current use OR 2.13, 95% CI 1.07–4.67) as was use of crack, cocaine, or heroin (current use OR 2.31, 95% CI 1.12–4.74).[46] Of course, it is difficult to interpret these data as most are cross-sectional and IVDU is a mode of transmission of the virus and opiates may be required as a treatment for severe pain.

In a recent systematic review of factors associated with physical activity among PLWHIV, bodily pain was a barrier to participation, as was depression.[52] Given the recognized importance of physical activity for health and well-being, this suggests that adequate treatment for pain could assist in health promotion for PLWHIV.

Psychological Factors

Psychological factors were not evaluated in many of the earlier studies, but where more recent studies have measured them, pain is strongly associated with different types of psychological ill-health and distress. For example, Rotheram-Borus[47] found that pain symptoms were significantly associated with depression, anxiety, and emotional distress. Richardson et al.[46] found that depression was highly significantly correlated with pain severity ($p < 0.0001$) and frequency ($p < 0.0001$). Five of the 26 studies included in the Parker systematic review considered psychological factors, all of which found an association between psychological distress (or mental illness) and pain.[42] Worse depression scores have been associated with more severe pain in two studies.[39,46] Peltzer et al.[43] were able to show that, among people with HIV associated sensory neuropathy, negative thoughts were associated with pain intensity, pain interference, and distress. Lawson et al.[28] found that, among 127/859 PLWHIV who reported chronic widespread pain (pain all over the body for at least 3 months), poor psychological health was associated with a four-fold higher risk (OR 3.97, 95% CI 2.15–7.32).

HIV Factors

The results of several studies have suggested that pain was more frequent with more advanced stages of HIV infection (stage III or IV or

Centre for Disease Control category C).[3,6,27,30,32,49] Richardson et al.[46] found that a CD4 count <200 × 10^9/L was significantly associated with pain severity (OR 2.22, 95% CI 1.4–3.5) and frequency (OR 1.84, 95% CI 1.2–2.9) in univariate analyses and that the relationship persisted in the multivariate model for pain severity (OR 2.08, 95% CI 1.22–3.51) but not frequency. Aouizerat et al.[2] reported similar findings with CD4 count. Frich and Borgbjerg[16] showed that the number of pain sites was inversely correlated with the CD4 count. Richardson et al.[46] also found that higher detectable viral load (>50,000 copies/mL) was significantly associated with frequency of pain (OR 1.88, 95% CI 1.2–3.1) but not pain severity in the univariate models, but that this relationship became nonsignificant in multivariate models. However, the relationship with disease severity has not been observed in all studies.[13,28,32,40] In a UK study, duration of time since diagnosis was an independent risk factor for pain in the final multivariable model (OR 1.17, 95% CI 1.03–1.32), even though this model also included age.[28]

The studies of Martin et al.,[32] Del Borgo et al.,[11] and Richardson et al.[46] demonstrated that the route of transmission of the HIV might also play a role, showing that the prevalence of pain was significantly higher among intravenous drug users as compared with nonintravenous drug users (85% vs. 71% respectively, $p < 0.05$), (72.9% vs. 50.6% respectively, $p = 0.008$), and (OR 1.83, 95% CI 1.13–2.97, $p = 0.01$), respectively, particularly among those in the mildest stage of HIV disease (asymptomatic).[32]

ANTIRETROVIRAL THERAPY AND PAIN

As described above, a number of the available pain studies were carried out in the pre-ART era. Even where a proportion of study subjects were receiving one or more ARTs, this was not considered as an independent risk factor in the earlier studies.[3,11] One of the earliest studies considering ART found less pain among ambulatory AIDS patients receiving ART as compared with those not receiving ART.[6] In contrast, Richardson et al.[46] included exposure to cART as an independent risk factor for pain and explored the effects of: no therapy; monotherapy; combination therapy; protease inhibitor (PI) based

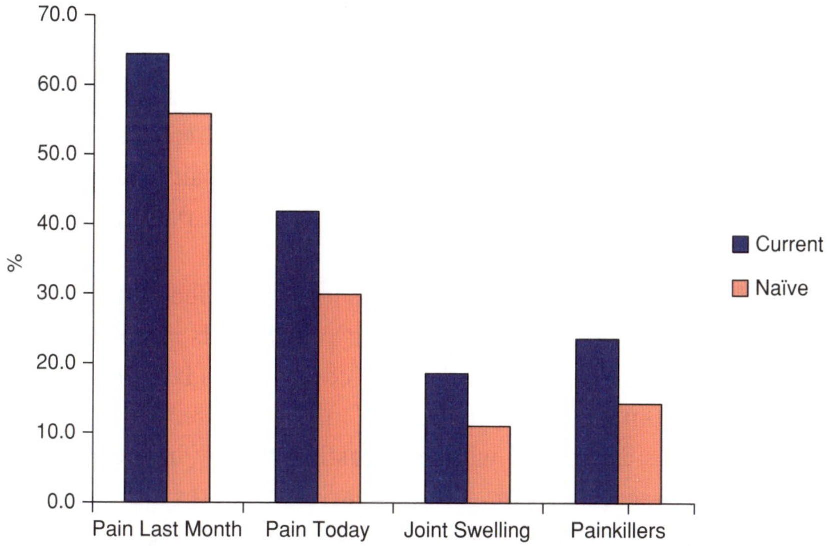

FIGURE 1-3 A comparison of pain experience among 859 PLWHIV comparing current users of ART with individuals who have never used ART.

ART; nonnucleoside reverse transcriptase inhibitor (NNRTI)-based ART; and finally ART including PI and NNRTI. None of these categories of ART were independently associated with frequency or severity of pain when compared with no treatment. Earlier this year, Wakeham et al.[55] reported on the symptom burden of PLWHIV and showed that the prevalence of pain reduced from 79% to 60% during the first year after initiation of ART. In contrast, among a cohort of patients with a mean duration since diagnosis of HIV of 6 years, ART users reported a higher prevalence of pain today and over the past month, more use of analgesia for pain and more swollen joints than individuals naïve to ART (Fig. 1-3).[28]

A clinical trial of 336 patients who had commenced ART 4 months previously including 1 PI (mostly indinavir) + 2 NRTIs reported that 32.1% subjects had experienced muscular pain at least once in the last month and 12.8% reported that they had experienced "distressing muscular pains."[14] Including 109 HIV-infected adults on ART, Johnson et al.[23] evaluated the prevalence and impact of 38 different symptoms and found that 79% reported stiff or painful joints and 77% aching muscles during the past 1 month of ART. After fatigue, these were, respectively, the second and third most frequently reported symptoms, more common than diarrhea, neuropathy and "feeling depressed." When ranked for the most bothersome symptoms, stiff or painful joints were ranked among the four most bothersome symptoms.[23] In contrast, other investigators reported lower pain intensity scores and more transient, rather than chronic, pain in 41 patients after treatment with cART.[8]

In clinical trials of PIs among naive HIV-infected patients and non-infected patients as postexposure prophylaxis, symptoms of muscle pain and joint pain are relatively commonly (10% to 30% incidence) reported but usually described as "mild" and "self-limiting."[7,14] Current PI use was associated with pain lasting >1 day in the past month in a UK cross-sectional survey in univariate analyses although the association was not robust to adjustment for other risk factors.[28] Interestingly, PIs were found associated with pain in another study of female HIV patients.[46] PIs have also been found associated with painful neuropathy[15] but more research is required to ascertain whether any individual drug or group of ART is associated with pain and what mechanisms underlie this association.

IMPACT OF PAIN IN HIV

Pain intensity has been measured in a range of different studies but with some variability in approach. However, where a standardized approach has been used, the pain reported by PLWHIV is of moderate-to-severe intensity. At this level of intensity, it is well recognized that pain has significant impact on ability to function and quality of life. This is borne out by the results of one study, in which 60% to 70% of those with pain reported that it interfered severely with aspects of their daily lives.[34] Another study found that 88% of patients in pain had at least one impairment in their daily life affecting activities including relaxing, sleeping, and walking.[3] In their study, Larue et al.[27] found that patients with significant pain reported poorer quality of life than patients without pain. Merlin et al.[36] reported that pain in HIV patients was associated with a 10-fold greater risk of impaired physical function, even after adjusting for mood, age, and substance abuse. In a South African study, PLWHIV described their pain as "frightening, unbearable, and intense" suggesting that the pain experience has emotional as well as physical impacts.[31] In their systematic review, Parker et al.[42] found that 9/28 studies reported the effects of pain on function and found a wide range of pain interfering with activity, as low as no interference among an urban population in South Africa through to moderate interference described by a USA sample.

HEALTHCARE UTILIZATION DUE TO PAIN IN HIV

The results from one UK cohort study would suggest that pain results in significant additional healthcare utilization.[28] Among 859 PLWHIV, they found a mean pain severity score of 5.1/10 and that, among those in pain, 28% had seen their primary healthcare provider about their pain, 9% had attended A&E, 23% were taking analgesics most days, and 18% of those currently employed had taken sickness absence that they attributed to their pain. Johnson et al.[22] studied HIV-positive patients attending a pain management service and found that most patients presented with chronic pain diagnoses, for example, spinal stenosis, degenerative disc disease, or neuropathy and found that pain clinic involvement reduced the need for attendance for emergency care. Jiao et al.[21] explored the impact of "chronic pain" conditions among PLWHIV, finding that 40% of 638 patients fulfilled criteria for one or more chronic pain conditions, among whom women, older patients, patients with greater burdens of medical illness, and psychiatric and substance misuse comorbidities were disproportionately represented. After controlling for overall health status, HIV patients with chronic pain required significantly more healthcare than those without.

MECHANISMS OF PAIN IN HIV

There has been limited research to date into the mechanisms of pain in HIV. It appears that HIV-related pain has both nociceptive and neuropathic components.[9] The sources of pain in HIV have been broadly characterized as: caused by the infection *per se*; consequential of immunosuppression; medication toxicity (ART and others); procedural pain; physical painful symptoms from depression and pain unrelated to HIV infection.[19] Potentially interesting new insight came from two recent studies. In the first, Goodin et al.[17] demonstrated that PLWHIV with detectable viral loads demonstrated significantly lower pain thresholds for mechanical stimuli and lower pain thresholds as compared with PLWHIV without detectable viral loads and healthy controls. This research may suggest that a detectable viral load may be able to sensitize PLWHIV to pain but further research is required. The second, by Merlin et al.,[37] found increased levels of Interleukin-1β (IL-1β) among PLWHIV with chronic pain as compared with PLWHIV without chronic pain. Clearly, as a cross-sectional relationship, it is as yet unknown whether this is cause of effect but these findings offer new avenues for research into pain mechanisms in HIV.

TREATMENT OF PAIN IN HIV

Going back to the very earliest studies of pain in HIV, there has been evidence of underestimation of pain in HIV and undertreatment. For example, one study evaluated response to analgesia in their cohort of patients and found that 40% were not prescribed any analgesia and that those receiving analgesics reported only 65% improvement from therapy. Similarly, 57% of those reporting pain in a French study did not receive any analgesia and only 22% were prescribed at least weak opioids.[27] This study also aimed to quantify the underestimation of pain by physicians by comparing the estimated pain scores of the physicians with those of the patients and found that the physicians underestimated pain in 52% of cases.[27] Underestimation was much more likely in patients with severe or moderate pain than those with mild pain and was less likely when the patient was perceived to be depressed or the doctor could not identify the source of pain. Rates of undertreatment appear to be similar in resource-poor countries[24]; for example, in a Nigerian study, 60% of patients reporting pain were receiving no treatment,[54] a figure similar to the 73% reporting no treatment in a South Indian study.[40] According to Breitbart, women and people with lower educational attainment were more likely to have their pain undertreated.[6] This may be because such patients are fearful of being thought difficult if they report their symptoms although some patients express concern that healthcare providers do not appear to take their pain symptoms seriously. Another cause of undertreatment, at least in clinics in resource-rich countries, may result from fear of addiction by patients and healthcare providers.[31]

Six studies in Parker et al.'s[42] systematic review reported on the adequacy of pain management using the standardized methods based upon the Pain Management Index. In all six studies, the majority of patients reported inadequate pharmacologic pain management.

With the exception of sensory neuropathy, there is a dearth of information on the efficacy of available analgesics in most HIV-related pain. Several opioid analgesics including morphine, codeine, hydrocodone, and fentanyl have potential interactions with some ART.[50] Moreover, opioid treatment is complex in this patient group with a high incidence of substance abuse. There is an urgent need for placebo-controlled trials of pharmacologic treatments in PLWHIV taking and not taking ART. Where placebo-controlled trials have been performed (for sensory neuropathy), results have been generally disappointing[12] with the exception of high-dose capsaicin patches.[45] Moreover, given the strong relationship between depression and other mental health pathologies and pain, controlled trials of psychosocial interventions, physical therapies, and complementary and alternative approaches including acupuncture, cognitive behavioral therapy, and educational interventions[35] are also urgently required.

In the absence of evidence, the recommended approach is to follow the WHO analgesic ladder, even in the absence of validation studies, even though this approach has known limitations in chronic HIV-associated pain.[26] It is clear that a biopsychosocial approach is indicated in this group of patients and that the pain is not viewed in isolation but rather in conjunction with optimization of virologic control and recognition and treatment of underlying secondary complications and side-effects of ART.

CONCLUSION

Pain is a common comorbidity of HIV, often affecting more than one anatomical site and frequently associated with moderate-to-severe functional impact. There does not appear to be much evidence that rates of pain have been attenuated by the advent of ART and it is unclear if ART causes pain. Risk factors for pain may include older age, female gender, poorer socioeconomic status, psychological distress, duration, and stage and severity of HIV infection. There are, however, too few data to be clear about the role of ethnicity, mode of transmission of infection, use of illicit substances, and whether any specific drug or group or regimen of ART affects the risk of pain. There is, however, consistent evidence of undertreatment of pain in HIV and more research is required in this area.

REFERENCES

1. Aigner CJ, Gritz ER, Tami-Maury I, et al. The role of pain in quitting among human immunodeficiency virus (HIV)-positive smokers enrolled in a smoking cessation trial. *Subst Abus*. 2017;38:249–252.
2. Aouizerat BE, Miaskowski CA, Gay C, et al. Risk factors and symptoms associated with pain in HIV-infected adults. *J Assoc Nurses AIDS Care*. 2010;21:125–133.
3. Bernard N, Spira R, Ybanez S, et al. Prevalence and underestimation of pain in HIV-infected patients by physicians: a cross-sectional study in a day care hospital. *AIDS*. 1999;13:293–295.
4. Bouhassira D. Pain from AIDS (adult). *Dev Sante*. 1997;(131):24–25.
5. Boyer V, Vilotitch A, Marcellin F, Demoulin B, Dray-Spira R, Spire B; ANRS-VESPA2 Study Group. Self-reported bothersome symptoms across different socioepidemiological groups of people living with HIV attending French hospitals: results from the ANRS-VESPA2 Survey. *J Pain Symptom Manage*. 2017;54:110–119.
6. Breitbart W, McDonald MV, Rosenfeld B, et al. Pain in ambulatory AIDS patients. I: pain characteristics and medical correlates. *Pain*. 1996;68:315–321.
7. Cahn P, Montaner J, Junod P, et al. Pilot, randomized study assessing safety, tolerability and efficacy of simplified LPV/r maintenance therapy in HIV patients on the 1st PI-based regimen. *PLoS One*. 2011;6:e23726.
8. Cervia LD, McGowan JP, Weseley AJ. Clinical and demographic variables related to pain in HIV-infected individuals treated with effective, combination antiretroviral therapy (cART). *Pain Med*. 2010;11:498–503.
9. Collins K, Harding R. Improving HIV management in sub-Saharan Africa. How much palliative care is needed? *AIDS Care*. 2007;19:1304–1306.

10. Crock EA, Miller C, McKenzie R, et al. Emerging needs of people living with HIV receiving community-based nursing in an Australian setting. *J Assoc Nurses AIDS Care*. 2017;28:644–658.

11. Del Borgo C, Izzi I, Chiarotti F, et al. Multidimensional aspects of pain in HIV-infected individuals. *AIDS Patient Care STDS*. 2001;15:95–102.

12. Dinat N, Marinda E, Moch S, Rice AS, Kamerman PR. Randomised, double-blind, crossover trial of amitryptilene for analgesia in painful HIV-associated sensory neuropathy, *PLoS One*. 2015;10:e0126297.

13. Dobalian A, Tsao JC, Duncan RP. Pain and the use of outpatient services among patients with HIV: results from a nationally representative survey. *Med Care*. 2004; 42:129–138.

14. Duran S, Spire B, Raffi F, et al. Self-reported symptoms after initiation of a protease inhibitor in HIV-infected patients and their impact on adherence to HAART. *HIV Clin Trials*. 2001;2:38–45.

15. Evans SR, Ellis RJ, Chen H, et al. Peripheral neuropathy in HIV: prevalence and risk factors. *AIDS*. 2011;25:919–928.

16. Frich LM, Borgbjerg FM. Pain and pain treatment in AIDS patients: a longitudinal study. *J Pain Symptom Manage*. 2000;19:339–347.

17. Goodin BR, Owens MA, Yessick LR, et al. Detectable viral load may be associated with increased pain sensitivity in persons living with HIV: preliminary findings. *Pain Med*. 2017;18:2289–2295.

18. Hansen L, Penko J, Guzman D, Bangsberg DR, Miaskowski C, Kushel MB. Aberrant behaviors with prescription opioids and problem drug use history in a community-based cohort of HIV-infected individuals. *J Pain Symptom Manage*. 2011;42:893–902.

19. Hewitt DJ, McDonald M, Portenoy RK, Rosenfeld B, Passik S, Breitbart W. Pain syndromes and etiologies in ambulatory AIDS patients. *Pain*. 1997;70:117–123.

20. Hitchcock SA, Meyer HP, Gwyther E. Neuropathic pain in AIDS patients prior to antiretroviral therapy. *S Afr Med J*. 2008;98:889–892.

21. Jiao JM, So E, Jebakumar J, George MC, Simpson DM, Robinson-Papp J. Chronic pain disorders in HIV primary care: clinical characteristics and association with healthcare utilization. *Pain*. 2016;157:931–937.

22. Johnson A, Condon KD, Mapas-Dimaya AC, et al. Report of an HIV clinic-based pain management program and utilisation of health status and health service by HIV patients. *J Opioid Manag*. 2012;8:17–27.

23. Johnson MO, Stallworth T, Neilands TB. The drugs or the disease? Causal attributions of symptoms held by HIV-positive adults on HAART. *AIDS Behav*. 2003;7: 109–117.

24. Kamerman PR, Mitchell D. Current perspectives on HIV-related pain and its management: insights from sub-Saharan Africa. *Pain Manag.* 2011;1:587–596.

25. Kelleher P, Cox S, McKeogh M. HIV infection: the spectrum of symptoms and disease in male and female patients attending a London hospice. *Palliat Med.* 1997;11: 152–158.

26. Koeppe J, Armon C, Lyda K, Nielsen C, Johnson S. Ongoing pain despite aggressive opioid pain management among persons with HIV. *Clin J Pain.* 2010;26:190–198.

27. Larue F, Fontaine A, Colleau SM. Underestimation and under treatment of pain in HIV disease: multicentre study. *BMJ.* 1997;314:23–28.

28. Lawson E, Sabin C, Perry N, et al. Is HIV painful? An epidemiologic study of the prevalence and risk factors for pain in HIV-infected patients. *Clin J Pain.* 2015;31:813–819.

29. Lebovits AH, Lefkowitz M, McCarthy D, et al. The prevalence and management of pain in patients with AIDS: a review of 134 cases. *Clin J Pain.* 1989;5:245–248.

30. Lolekha R, Chanthavanich P, Limkittikul K, Luangxay K, Chotpitayasunodh T, Newman CJ. Pain: a common symptom in human immunodeficiency virus-infected Thai children. *Acta Paediatr.* 2004;93:891–898.

31. Maree JE, Dreyer Wright SC, Makua MR. The management of HIV- and AIDS-related pain in a primary health clinic in Tshwane, South Africa. *Pain Manag Nurs.* 2013;14:94–101.

32. Martin C, Pehrsson P, Östenberg A, Sönnerborg A, Hansson P. Pain in ambulatory HIV-infected patients with and without intravenous drug use. *Eur J Pain.* 1999;3:157–164.

33. May MT, Vehreschild JJ, Trickey A, et al. Mortality according to CD4 count at start of combination antiretroviral therapy among HIV-infected patients followed for up to 15 years after start of treatment: collaborative cohort study. *Clin Infect Dis.* 2016; 62:1571–1577.

34. McCormack JP, Li R, Zarowny D, Singer J. Inadequate treatment of pain in ambulatory HIV patients. *Clin J Pain.* 1993;9:279–283.

35. Mello A, Gravel T. HIV pain management challenges and alternative therapies. *Nursing.* 2017;47:67–70. Available from www.Nursing 2017.com (April 2017). Accessed online (August 2017).

36. Merlin JS, Westfall AO, Chamot E, et al. Pain is independently associated with impaired physical function in HIV-infected patients. *Pain Med.* 2013;14:1985–1993.

37. Merlin JS, Westfall AO, Heath SL, et al. Brief report: IL-1β levels are associated with chronic multisite pain in people living with HIV. *J Acquir Immune Defic Syndr.* 2017;75:e99–e103.

38. Merlin JS, Westfall AO, Raper JL, et al. Pain, mood, substance abuse in HIV: implications for clinic visit utilisation, ART adherence and virologic failure. *J Acquir Immune Defic Syndr*. 2012;61:164–170.

39. Miaskowski C, Penko JM, Guzman D, Mattson JE, Bangsberg DR, Kushel MB. Occurrence and characteristics of chronic pain in a community-based cohort of indigent adults living with HIV infection. *J Pain*. 2011;12:1004–1016.

40. Nair SN, Mary TR, Prarthana S, Harrison P. Prevalence of pain in patients with HIV/AIDS: a cross-sectional survey in a South Indian state. *Indian J Palliat Care*. 2009;15:67–70.

41. Norval DA. Symptoms and sites of pain experienced by AIDS patients. *S Afr Med J*. 2004;94:450–454.

42. Parker R, Stein DJ, Jelsma J. Pain in people living with HIV/AIDS: a systematic review. *J Int AIDS Soc*. 2014;17:18719.

43. Peltzer K, Preez NF, Ramlagan S, Fomundam H. Use of traditional complementary and alternative medicine for HIV patients in Kwazulu-Natal, South Africa. *BMC Public Health*. 2008;8:255.

44. Penfold J, Clark AJ. Pain syndromes in HIV infection. *Can J Anaesth*. 1992;39:724–730.

45. Phillips TJ, Cherry CL, Cox S, Marshall SJ, Rice AS. Pharmacological treatment of HIV-associated sensory neuropathy: a systematic review and meta-analysis of randomised controlled trials. *PLoS One*. 2010;5:E14433.

46. Richardson JL, Heikes B, Karim R, Weber K, Anastos K, Young M. Experience of pain among women with advanced HIV disease. *AIDS Patient Care STDS*. 2009;23:503–511.

47. Rotheram-Borus MJ. Variations in perceived pain associated with emotional distress and social identity in AIDS. *AIDS Patient Care STDS*. 2000;14:659–665.

48. Schofferman J. Care of the terminally ill person with AIDS. *Int Ophthalmol Clin*. 1989;29:127–130.

49. Singer EJ, Zorilla C, Fahy-Chandon B, Chi S, Syndulko K, Tourtellotte WW. Painful symptoms reported by ambulatory HIV-infected men in a longitudinal study. *Pain*. 1993;54:15–19.

50. University of Liverpool HIV drug interactions 2017. Available from www.hiv- druginteractions.org/checker

51. UN Joint Programme on HIV/AIDS. Global Report: UN AIDS report on the global AIDS epidemic 2013. United Nations, Geneva (2013 November). Available from http://www.unaids.org/en/resources/campaigns/globalreport2013/globalreport/

52. Vancampfort D, Mugisha J, Richards J, De Hert M, Probst M, Stubbs B. Physical activity correlates in people living with HIV/AIDS: a systematic review of 45 studies. *Disabil Rehabil*. 2018;40:1618–1629.

53. Verma S, Estanislao L, Simpson D. HIV-associated neuropathic pain: epidemiology, pathophysiology and management. *CNS Drugs*. 2005;19:325–334.

54. Wahab KW, Salami AK. Pain as a symptom in patients living with HIV/AIDS seen at the outpatient clinic of a Nigerian tertiary hospital. *J Int Assoc Physicians AIDS Care (Chic)*. 2011;10:35–39.

55. Wakeham K, Harding R, Levin J, Parkes-Ratanshi R, Kamali A, Lalloo DG. The impact of antiretroviral therapy on symptom burden among HIV outpatients with low CD4 count in rural Uganda: nested longitudinal cohort study. *BMC Palliat Care*. 2017;17:8.

56. Wilson NL, Azuero A, Vance DE, et al. Identifying symptom patterns in people living with HIV Disease. *J Assoc Nurses AIDS Care*. 2016;27:121–132.

CHAPTER 2

Management of Pain in Iatrogenic Nerve Injury

Sudheesh Ramachandran and Rajiv Midha

Iatrogenic injuries are, in their strictest sense, those inflicted by the physician. Unfortunately, iatrogenic peripheral nerve injuries (PNIs) are exceedingly common. Lack of adequate knowledge of peripheral nerve anatomy and the ubiquitous nature of peripheral nerves contributes to the relatively high frequency of nerve injury in these settings. Some of the possible causes include direct damage during surgery; pressure or traction because of positioning during anesthesia; injection of neurotoxic substances; compression by a hematoma secondary to drawing blood or through anticoagulation; compression from tourniquet, dressings, casts, or orthotic devices; and radiation-induced damage. In a series by Kretschmer et al.,[26] iatrogenic nerve injuries accounted for 17.4% of all traumatic nerve injuries, of which 94% was associated with a surgical procedure. Akin to any nerve injury, iatrogenic nerve injuries also result in pain, in addition to motor deficits and sensory loss.

Pain is a frequent complaint after PNI, the cause of which is usually multifactorial.[9] Owing to this, the management of pain in such settings is extremely challenging. Basically, two types of pain are seen—neuropathic and nonneuropathic—which stems from a constellation of factors such as the presence of neuromas, deafferentation, autonomic disturbances, and even disuse related swelling, joint stiffness along with shortening and fibrosis of muscles and tendons. The character of pain (crushing, burning, and paresthetic), location, aggravating/relieving factors, and response to medication often yields an accurate diagnosis which may be instrumental in successful management. In this chapter, we briefly review the etiopathology of neuropathic pain (NP) and management strategies for optimal outcome.

PATHOPHYSIOLOGY

Peripheral NP can be categorized into spontaneous pain (stimulus independent) or stimulus hypersensitivity secondary to damage to or alteration in the sensory neurons (stimulus dependent).[47] Following injury, an abnormal milieu of inflammatory mediators and cytokines can sensitize the nociceptor terminals such that they respond to even normal stimuli. The altered chemical microenvironment changes the function, chemistry, or even survival of cells. Loss of cells or axons subsequently reduces sensibility and induces changes in the surviving neurons. Schwann cell dedifferentiation initiated by nerve injury leads to the synthesis of growth factors and other chemical mediators, as opposed to maintaining myelin integrity, which have profound effects on neighboring intact and injured neurons.

The NP experience is the result of abnormal neurotransmission in the primary sensory neurons along with central/peripheral sensitization and sympathetic sprouting.[47] Spontaneous activity in nociceptor C fibers is known to give rise to persistent burning pain and sensitization of dorsal horn neurons. Also, similar activity in the large myelinated A fibers leads to paresthesias, dysesthesias, and pain. Both of them contribute to stimulus-independent pain which is one of the hallmarks of NP. On the contrary, the key features of stimulus-dependent pain are hyperalgesia and allodynia. Hyperalgesia is an increased pain response to a normally suprathreshold noxious stimulus and is the result of abnormal processing of nociceptor input whereas allodynia is the sensation of pain elicited by a nonnoxious stimulus and is mainly produced in two ways: by the action of low-threshold myelinated a beta fibers on an altered central nervous system and by a reduction in the threshold of nociceptor terminals in the periphery. Stimulus hyperalgesia can be caused by mechanical, thermal, or chemical stimuli.

Mechanistic Basis of Peripheral Neuropathic Pain

There are two types of sodium channels found in sensory neurons—those which are sensitive to tetrodotoxin (a potent pufferfish toxin) and those which are not. The former is present in all sensory neurons and is responsible for initiation of action potential whereas the latter is present only on nociceptor neurons.[33] Following nerve injury, both types of channels begin to accumulate in the axon at the neuroma site and along the length of axon resulting in foci of hyperexcitability and ectopic action potential discharge in the axon and cell body of injured neurons.[12] This causes the characteristic stimulus-independent pain. In partial nerve injury, alpha-adrenoceptors are overexpressed in injured and uninjured neurons, thus rendering them sensitive to circulating catecholamines and noradrenaline released from postganglionic sympathetic terminals.[47] This creates an abnormal phenomenon in which the sensory fibers are coactivated with sympathetic activity. This would explain the efficacy of sympathetic blockade in alleviation of symptoms in a minority of patients. In addition to the spontaneous activity in primary sensory neurons, decreased inhibitory GABAergic activity on primary sensory neurons and dorsal horns is one of the key reasons for stimulus independent pain. An improved understanding of the role of inhibitory neurotransmitters in the pathogenesis of pain has led to the introduction of Gabapentin, a GABA inhibitor, for alleviation of NP. Transcutaneous electrical nerve stimulation (TENS) is also known to upregulate the inhibitory neurotransmission.

Stimulus evoked pain is mostly manifested as mechanical hyperalgesia. Glutamic acid, which is an excitatory neurotransmitter, is the main mediator of this response. Activation of nociceptors causes the release of glutamate from central terminals that acts on the ionotropic glutamate receptor amino-3-hydroxy 5-methylisoxazole-4-proprionic acid (AMPA) and *N*-methyl-D-aspartate (NMDA) postsynaptically to cause a rapid depolarization in dorsal horn neurons, initiating an action potential if threshold is reached. Substance P acts on neurokinin I receptors, prolonging depolarization, increasing intracellular concentrations of calcium and thus increasing excitability, and thereby works in concert with glutamate activity. Interestingly, the nociceptive input to the dorsal horn increases the excitability of neuronal membranes which changes the way neurons respond to subsequent inputs. This phenomenon is termed central sensitization. It manifests in three different ways: (1) enlargement of the area in the periphery where a stimulus will activate neurons; (2) increased response to a suprathreshold input; and (3) previously subthreshold inputs reaching threshold thus initiating action potential discharge. These features mediated by A beta fibers, manifested as hypersensitivity to pain and also as the spread of pain beyond the territory of the affected nerve, which are hallmarks of central sensitization.[47]

CAUSES OF IATROGENIC NERVE INJURIES

Iatrogenic PNIs can occur in a variety of ways which mainly include anesthetic/surgical complications and improper operative positioning. Other causes are tourniquets, dressings, casts, orthotic devices, and radiation.[27,44]

Positioning related injuries comprise a substantial portion of iatrogenic nerve injuries. These injuries are usually secondary to stretch or compression. For instance, brachial plexus injuries are known to occur with arm hyperabduction, arm abduction with lateral flexion of the head to the contralateral side, or caudal pressure to the shoulder by the shoulder brace used in the Trendelenburg position.[46] Ulnar nerve injuries were frequently associated with improper padding and/or positioning of the elbow. The most important site of injury for radial nerve was the mid posterior arm when the arm was left unpadded and hanging at the edge of the table. Hanging the unpadded, pronated arm off the table carries the risk of median nerve injury. Anesthetic complications include nerve damage following injections such as those secondary to local anesthetic infiltration or injection of neurotoxic drugs, axillary region block, interscalene block, or during percutaneous central venous catheterization of the subclavian or internal jugular vein.[23]

Surgical complications contribute to a major portion of iatrogenic PNI. During surgery, nerves can be inadvertently cut, particularly when they are not clearly exposed in the operative field or when not properly identified and mistaken for a tendon or vessel. They also can be crushed, tied off, penetrated, or twisted during implantation or removal of osteosynthetic devices. There have been many reports of nerve injury during removal of a nerve sheath tumor or lymph nodes. For instance, the spinal accessory nerve is known to be injured during lymph node biopsies involving neck dissections of the posterior triangle. It is not uncommon among surgeons to have insufficient knowledge regarding aberrant anatomic course of peripheral nerves. This is one of the crucial factors contributing to iatrogenic nerve injuries.

It is important to note that some surgical procedures are more frequently associated with inadvertent nerve damage. These include osteosynthesis and osteotomies, arthrodesis, lymph node biopsy in the posterior triangle of the neck, carpal tunnel syndrome surgery, varicose vein surgery, Baker cyst excision, and inguinal herniorrhaphy. Also, certain high-risk sites have been described with regard to iatrogenic nerve injury. These include carpal tunnel, wrist, posterior triangle of the neck, and popliteal fossa where the nerves are superficial and in close proximity to the surgical target such as lymph node or Baker cyst. The ulnar nerve at the cubital tunnel and the peroneal nerve at the neck of fibula are particularly vulnerable to trauma during improper surgical positioning or application of casts due to their superficial location.

Studies have also shown that certain peripheral nerves have a higher risk of inadvertent injury perioperatively. In the largest series of 340 patients with iatrogenic nerve injuries published to date, the following were the most common nerves involved in the descending order: median nerve, accessory nerve, radial nerve, common peroneal nerve, ulnar nerve, and femoral nerve.[2,25,26] As mentioned earlier, the carpal tunnel release was the most common cause for iatrogenic median nerve injury. In this series, the risk appeared to be less with an endoscopic approach and the open approach was found to be more morbid when the surgeon tried to mimic the endoscopic approach using a mini-incision resulting in improper visualization of relevant surgical anatomy, particularly the flexor retinaculum. However, many authors have reported that, although the endoscopic approach is associated with lesser pain, the incidence of reversible postoperative nerve injury was high compared to open approach.[38,49]

APPROACH TO IATROGENIC NERVE INJURIES

Anesthetic or surgical complications should be evident in the immediate postoperative period. However, it is not infrequent to miss such a complication during the course of hospitalization. For instance, studies have shown that following total hip and knee replacements, only 77% to 90% of the sensorimotor and 20% of the sensory complications were recorded during the procedural hospitalization.[21] This is mainly due to certain barriers which prevent early recognition of PNI.[42] These include:

1. Sedation
2. Postoperative pain or analgesics
3. Regional anesthesia
4. Patient perioperative naivety/uncertainty
5. Postoperative activity restrictions
6. Dressings, drains, and casts.

It is also important to know about the risk factors that are potentially associated with iatrogenic PNI. Male sex; elderly age; extremes of body habitus; positive smoking status; and pre-existing peripheral nerve pathology such as diabetes, hereditary peripheral neuropathy, and peripheral vascular disease are known to create a predisposition for nerve damage. Casscells et al.[8] reported postoperative ulnar neuropathy in 26% of their patients who underwent open heart surgery, all of whom were known to have preoperative conduction slowing across the elbow. It is also imperative to gather adequate perioperative information. This has paramount diagnostic and therapeutic implications. These include history of neurologic symptoms with needle placement, prolonged tourniquet time, concomitant sedation with regional block, hypothermia, and prolonged hospitalization. According to the International Association for the Study of Pain (IASP), the diagnostic workup of a patient with nerve injury should include detailed medical history, review of systems and a thorough physical and neurologic examination. The medical history should provide important information about the onset, distribution, and quality of pain (electric shooting, aching, and burning).

The distribution of neurologic deficit/symptom has to be correlated with the site of anesthesia or surgery. It is important to determine whether the deficit/symptom is consistent with a mononeuropathy, plexopathy, or within the field of peripheral nerve blockade. Reversible causes of neurologic impairment such as hematoma or inflammation should be ruled out at the outset. It is prudent to obtain an early neurologic consultation if the deficits are severe, progressive, functionally disabling, multifocal, or difficult to localize. Observation is appropriate if the symptoms are purely sensory or mild in nature as most of these are self-limiting.

Clinical uncertainties could be confirmed using electrophysiologic studies. These studies help to confirm the suspected neurogenic process, localization, and characterization of the condition. The utility of early studies (before 3 weeks) is very limited as axonal damage is not very evident until Wallerian degeneration has occurred and there has been muscle denervation. Conduction block or focal slowing on nerve conduction velocity (NCV) is caused by focal demyelination secondary to compression suggestive of neurapraxia. Higher grades of injury are characterized by loss of amplitude and increase in latency. Serial electrophysiologic tests will be valuable in differentiating between axonotmesis and neurotmesis as only the former show evidence of reinnervation on early electromyography (EMG) studies. Magnetic resonance imaging (MRI) or ultrasonography (USG) can be helpful both in the acute and chronic stage for identifying structural lesions such as hematoma or neuroma. MRI appearance of end bulb and neuroma in continuity (NIC) type neuromas are similar and have a signal which is isointense to skeletal muscles on T1. Owing to a combination of fascicles, intralesional hemorrhage, and fibrosis, they are heterogeneous on fluid-sensitive sequences. Lack of contrast enhancement is helpful in differentiating neuromas from nerve sheath tumors.

It is extremely important to distinguish NP from non–nerve-related pain in the setting of PNI as it has significant therapeutic implications. Several published screening tools such as The Leeds Assessment of Neuropathic Symptoms and Signs (LANSS),[4] Neuropathic Pain Questionnaire (NPQ),[24] Douleur Neuropathique 4 Questions,[6] painDETECT,[15] and ID Pain[35] are immensely helpful in identifying NP. Additional tools are available to quantify the severity of NP and assess treatment response. These include the Neuropathic Pain Scale, Neuropathic Pain Symptom Inventory, and Short-Form McGill Pain Questionnaire 2.[22]

DIFFERENTIAL DIAGNOSIS OF PAIN

Neuropathic Pain

The IASP defines NP as the pain directly resulting from a lesion or disease affecting the somatosensory system.[40] As mentioned earlier, it can be spontaneous or driven by stimuli.[16] NP has a phenotype that is usually quite distinct from the pain arising from soft tissue injury usually manifesting as allodynia, in which the pain is induced by an innocuous stimulus such as light touch, or hyperalgesia where there is an exaggerated response to a painful stimulus. Other descriptors typically used by patients include burning, pins and needles, shooting, or electrical type sensation. When associated with a distinct past history of nerve injury, the physician should have a low threshold for a diagnosis of NP.

Postsurgical Inflammatory Neuropathy

The classic presentation of this entity includes severe pain hours to weeks (up to 30 days) after a stressor such as anesthesia or surgery, in a territory unrelated to them.[1,36] Perioperative sedation and analgesia is a huge deterrent to early diagnosis. As the pain spontaneously improves, weakness becomes apparent which can be multifocal or diffuse. Localized inflammation or ischemia is known to be cause of this condition; however, it is still not entirely clear why nonoperated nerves are affected. Histology shows neuronal lymphocytic infiltration with microvasculitis.[36] The prognosis is generally good as this condition is self-limiting. Patients with a multifocal or difficult-to-localize postoperative deficit, associated severe pain disproportionate to the expected perioperative course, progressive deficits, or deficits developing after a period of documented return to neurologic baseline should be evaluated for the possibility of a postsurgical inflammatory neuropathy with early neurologic consultation.

Complex Regional Pain Syndrome

Complex regional pain syndrome (CRPS) is a severe variant of NP and cannot be overlooked in any discussion on neurogenic pain. It is characterized by an inexplicable, disproportionately severe pain associated with autonomic disturbances, classically manifested as changes in blood flow, disturbed perception of cold and warmth, sudomotor activity, edema, and pigmentation changes.[20] CRPS type 1 is not associated with an identifiable nerve injury whereas type II is a result of detectable nerve injury. It is not uncommon for the onset of symptoms to be delayed by several weeks or months following injury. Although CRPS is a straightforward diagnosis, misdiagnosis of type II as type I is highly common because of missed nerve injuries, particularly when they are iatrogenic. An accurate diagnosis is extremely important, as CRPS type II pain syndromes are hard to treat without addressing the injured nerve.

Neuroma

PNIs occasionally result in neuromas which can give rise to maladaptive NP. Studies have shown that the incidence of symptomatic neuromas is around 3% to 5%.[37] They are abnormal conglomeration of axonal sprouts entrapped in scar tissue, not reaching their proximal or distal target.[30] They cause pain when there is mechanical traction, compression, chemical irritation, or development of ectopic ion channels. In clinical practice, they are suspected based on the above clinical features, or discovered incidentally on imaging or nerve repair. Trigger point injections or nerve blocks may aid in diagnosis.

Miscellaneous Pain Syndromes

Apart from those aforementioned, PNI is also known to cause the following pain syndromes:

1. Reinnervation pain: This is a type of hypersensitivity pain related to the process of muscle and cutaneous receptor re-innervation. It is characterized by lancinating, electrical, tingling, and/or shock like pain along the course of a nerve or within an affected muscle or skin, and usually occurs as a "new" pain later in the course, consistent with the time-course of nerve regeneration.
2. Avulsion pain: This is seen in iatrogenic brachial plexus injuries secondary to nerve root avulsion. It is characterized by a severe crushing, burning, or freezing pain usually experienced in the distal portion of an insensate limb.
3. Neuritis pain: As the name implies, this is caused by inflammation of a nerve segment. The pain is usually sharp, lancinating, or electrical in nature experienced in the distribution of the sensory nerve.
4. Musculoskeletal pain: This type of pain is often thought to be neurogenic, but arises from joint and muscle imbalance, muscle atrophy, shortening, and fibrosis; it may arise with Charcot joint. It is often described as a soreness or aching pain predominantly over the affected joints, muscles, and/or tendons.

MANAGEMENT OF PAIN

The treatment of pain following PNI is extremely challenging. As the reason for pain is often multifactorial, the therapy is multifaceted. The patient might have had very little communication regarding their symptom with the primary physician and often their expectations of full functional recovery are quite high. It is not uncommon among primary physicians to have underestimated the extent of neurologic insult. A thorough evaluation of pain should include neurologic, musculoskeletal, general system, and psychological evaluation along with an extensive history. Electrodiagnostic tests are helpful in pinpointing the location and also assessing the extent of injury. An extensive discussion with the concerned surgical staff; information regarding suspicious sutures, clips, or instrumentation; and concerns documented during intraoperative vascular, hemodynamic, and electrophysiologic monitoring are extremely beneficial. The pain clinician should be very careful regarding the manner in which information is divulged to the patient, not only for therapeutic and medicolegal reasons, but also to ensure that proper etiquette is maintained to preserve future relationships with referring physicians. NP is rarely cured but most patients experience satisfactory pain relief and better quality of life after appropriate therapy. The reasons for treatment failure includes inaccurate diagnosis, incorrect selection of treatment, lack of understanding of the mechanisms, and inappropriate management of comorbid conditions such as behavioral and psychiatric complications associated with chronic pain.

In any patient with suspected PNI, an ongoing reversible process causing neurologic impairment such as hematoma or inflammation should be ruled out at the outset. For instance, a retroperitoneal hematoma can cause lumbar plexopathy and perineural hematomas can present as mononeuropathy. When a bleeding complication is considered, urgent imaging (USG or computerized tomography [CT]) is strongly recommended. Reversal of anticoagulation should be followed by surgical evacuation, if necessary, in severe cases. It is also important to rule out the possibility of compartment syndrome. The neurologic evaluation should be performed and analyzed in the light of recent anesthetic/surgical procedure. It is critical to determine whether the deficits are concordant with the procedure site. If the deficits are consistent with a mononeuropathy at a common site of involvement (e.g., ulnar nerve at the cubital tunnel or peroneal nerve at the fibular head) or purely sensory in nature, close observation will suffice usually. In such instances, management is mainly comprised of PT/OT, rehab needs, pain management, and neurologic follow-up. If sufficient characterization and localization of the deficit is difficult, due to the various barriers mentioned earlier, an acute electrophysiologic study may be considered. This will be helpful in detecting neurapraxia; however, axonal damage cannot be identified until Wallerian degeneration and muscle denervation has occurred which typically takes 2 to 3 weeks. Apart from this, there are no strong indications to

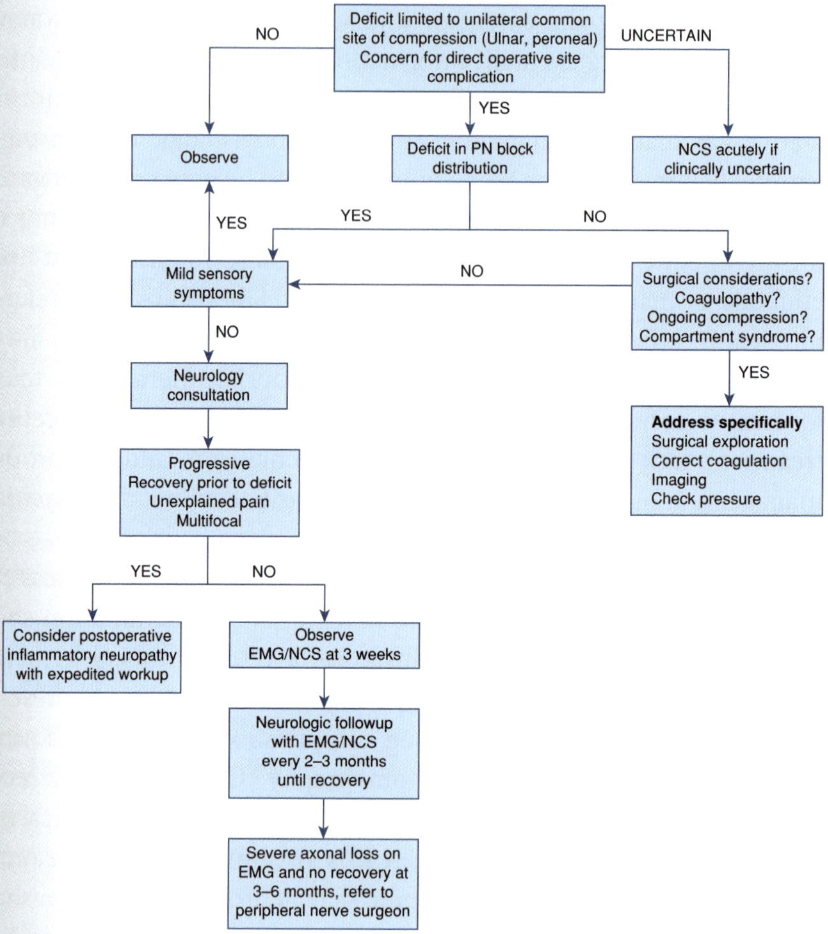

Courtesy: Watson JC, Huntoon MA. Neurologic Evaluation and Management of Perioperative Nerve Injury. Reg Anesth Pain Med. 2015;40(5):491-501.

FIGURE 2-1 Approach to iatrogenic perioperative nerve injury. EMG, electromyography; NCS, nerve conduction study; PN, peripheral nerve.

perform an acute electrophysiologic study. Early neurologic consultation is appropriate when the deficits are severe, functionally limiting, progressive, and difficult to localize (Fig. 2-1).

PHARMACOLOGIC MANAGEMENT

Following diagnosis, all patients with significant pain should be initiated on treatment using an evidence-based guideline for oral and topical medications (Neuropathic pain special interest group and European federation of Neurological Societies).[3,13,14] Many of these guidelines were formulated for painful diabetic neuropathy or postherpetic neuralgia; however, they are known to be effective for pain secondary to any cause including iatrogenic trauma. Current guidelines follow a tiered approach progressing from single first-line agents to multiple first-line agents, followed by second- and third-line agents when treatment goals are not met. First-line drugs include nortriptyline, desipramine (tricyclic antidepressants [TCA]), duloxetine (selective serotonin reuptake inhibitors [SSRIs]), anticonvulsants acting at the α-2-δ neuronal calcium channels (gabapentin and pregabalin), and topical 5% lidocaine. These drugs are generally safe but runs the risk of anticholinergic side effects, cardiac toxicity (TCAs), and serotonin syndrome (SSRI interaction with opioids). Opioids such as morphine, oxycodone, and tramadol constitute the second line. Constipation, nausea, and sedation are the most common adverse effects of these drugs. It is important to initiate treatment with low doses and gradually titrate based on clinical requirements. It is also important to consider the risk of substance abuse, particularly in patients with previous history or family history of abuse. Third-line drugs have much lower quality studies to support their use and also are known to contradict evidence from well-designed trials. This class includes certain antidepressant medications (e.g., bupropion, citalopram, and paroxetine), certain antiepileptic medications (e.g., carbamazepine, lamotrigine, oxcarbazepine, topiramate, and valproic acid), dextromethorphan, memantine, mexiletine, lacosamide, botulinum toxin, and topical low-concentration capsaicin.

NONPHARMACOLOGIC MANAGEMENT

Cognitive Behavioral Therapy

Medications often do not provide complete relief of NP. Therapeutic goals include not only pain relief, but also improved physical function, diminished psychological stress, and heightened overall quality of life. Hence addressing the psychological component of pain is key to optimal management. Providers can help patients by focusing on wellness behavior, functionality, and normal participation in activities. Pain catastrophization, which refers to exaggerating the degree and effect of pain experienced, is known to be a major predictor of poor response to pharmacotherapy and thus contributes significantly to greater disability and poor quality of life.[39] Cognitive behavioral therapy addresses this maladaptive behavior, thus helping patients to change their thoughts and emotions through training in coping skills.

Support Groups

They serve as an outlet for patients and also promotes patient's engagement in the treatment strategy. Interaction with other patients suffering in a similar fashion allows them to share coping techniques and provide positive reinforcement for improved functioning.

Interventional Blocks

Targeted blockade of an implicated nerve provides relief of pain in the specific dermatome. Generally, these are performed only in patients who have failed conservative management techniques due to risk of infection, bleeding, and potential nerve damage. Complications are infrequent under experienced hands. Peripheral nerve blocks are usually performed with local anesthetics and/or steroids. These blocks are often diagnostic and therapeutic. Neuralgias of the trunk or extremity such as meralgia paresthetica or inguinal neuralgia secondary to hernia repair can be easily targeted. The margin of safety is improved with image guidance such as fluoroscopy and USG in some locations such as intercostal neuralgia. Sympathetic nerve blocks are generally reserved for NP patients with CRPS. Stellate ganglion and lumbar sympathetic blocks are the commonly used blocks for upper- and lower-extremity pain, respectively. Some clinical features such as allodynia and hypoesthesia help to predict response to sympathetic blockade.[41]

Neurolysis

The major downside of nerve blocks with local anesthesia (LA) is that they provide only short-term relief. When coupled with radiofrequency (RF) or chemical neurolysis, they can provide lasting relief. However, there is a small chance of aggravation of symptoms with the aforementioned techniques. Pulsed radiofrequency (PRF) treatment uses intermittent high frequency current to ablate nerves. This technique uses a lower temperature (<42°C) compared to conventional RF ablation. PRF has high safety profile and can be used even on motor nerves without causing motor deficit.[7] Chemical neurolysis of sympathetic ganglia using alcohol, glycerol and phenol can alleviate regional pain. Potential complications of neurolysis include neurologic deficits, creation of painful neuromas, or neuritis. As mentioned earlier, image guidance has a huge influence on the success rate of nerve blocks. They are known to improve localization and precision of drug delivery. High-resolution USG has been used by many authors to guide injection for alleviation of pain due to neuromas. In a prospective study, Gruber et al.[18] reported good outcome in 82 patients who underwent ultrasound-guided chemical neurolysis using 80% phenol.

Neurostimulation

This includes TENS and spinal cord stimulation. TENS is a useful adjunct when conservative management fails. The mechanism is based on the gate control theory.[29] The input of the small afferent pain fibers on the dorsal horn is known to be inhibited with stimulation of large afferent fibers, thus closing the gate for further transmission. TENS is generally free of side effects. The spinal cord stimulator has been in use for decades and has proven to be an effective alternative. Deer et al.[10] showed 50% pain reduction with cervical spinal cord stimulation in a group of patients with chronic pain. Currently, they are mostly used in brachial plexus injuries. Potential complications include ineffective pain control, overstimulation, migration of leads, infection, dural puncture, CSF leak, or device malfunction requiring surgical removal or repositioning.

Surgical Management

Surgical intervention is recommended when pain following iatrogenic nerve injury is refractory to pharmacotherapeutic options. Recent evidence suggests that early nerve repair and grafting can yield satisfactory results. Bertelli and Ghizoni[5] demonstrated significant pain reduction following spinal nerve root grafting in brachial plexus avulsion injuries. Although surgery is not routinely recommended for CRPS, type II CRPS is known to improve with release or decompression of entrapped nerves. Dellon et al.[11] showed substantial reduction of pain due to CRPS, in a group of patients with lower-extremity injuries. Today, most authors recommend surgical intervention for refractory type II CRPS.

DREZ lesioning is an effective option for intractable NP or deafferentation pain. This procedure entails cauterization of the dorsal root entry zones to disrupt the peripheral nerve sensory inputs at the spinal cord level. This procedure is known to have lasting results on pain control. Haninec et al.,[19] in a study of 52 patients with brachial plexus injuries, demonstrated 75% pain reduction at 2-year follow-up. The complications of this procedure include ipsilateral leg motor or posterior column sensory modality dysfunction.

Selective ganglionectomy is a very effective option for intractable NP, particularly in the thoracic region. Dramatic symptomatic improvement has been reported by many authors without sensory loss, especially when only one ganglion was removed.[34,43,45] This therapeutic strategy is based on the fact that ectopic firing of the dorsal root ganglion is one of the fundamental causes of NP. A few authors believe that this procedure can result in the creation of NP. However, selective ganglionectomy, although safe and effective, does not provide lasting relief.[31] Recurrent pain outside the initially affected dermatome has been reported.

Resection of Neuromas

Neuromas should preferably be resected when they are painful. The resection of neuromas and repair with grafts is a very effective option. This restores the integrity of the nerve, eradicates the nociceptive focus, and guides the axons to their end organs. However, when such a reconstructive option is not feasible, the surgeon must try to place the neuroma in a friendlier environment. This is done by resecting the neuroma and placing the nerve stump deep to the skin in local bone or muscle.[17,28] It is prudent to mobilize this away from a joint in order to avoid traction. Studies have shown that surgical resection of neuroma is a better alternative to pharmacotherapy.[32,37] Alternatively, the neuromas can be resected and the gap between the stumps can be bridged using an autologous sural nerve graft.[28] Epineural flaps and epineural free grafts may be used for capping of nerve stumps with or without resection of nerve fascicles.[48]

Other therapeutic adjuncts include nonconventional techniques such as acupuncture, meditation, massage, cupping, movement therapies, yoga, tai chi, and reflexology.

CONCLUSIONS

Iatrogenic nerve injuries are, fortunately, not very common. Most injuries result in sensory symptoms which are often self-limiting and can be managed with patient reassurance, education, and scheduled follow-up to ensure symptomatic improvement. The management of pain secondary to nerve injury is extremely challenging. It is important to rule out an active, reversible cause at the outset by using appropriate investigations, and in select appropriate cases, offer surgical exploration and decompression. Early neurologic evaluation should be considered when the deficits are severe, progressive, and difficult to localize. Most cases can be managed with pharmacotherapy and surgery should be reserved only for refractory cases. A systematic tiered pain management approach and proactive rehabilitation can significantly improve patient function and quality of life.

REFERENCES

1. Ahn KS, Kopp SL, Watson JC, Scott KP, Trousdale RT, Hebl JR. Postsurgical inflammatory neuropathy. *Reg Anesth Pain Med.* 2011;36(4):403–405.
2. Antoniadis G, Kretschmer T, Pedro MT, Konig RW, Heinen CP, Richter HP. Iatrogenic nerve injuries: prevalence, diagnosis and treatment. *Dtsch Arztebl Int.* 2014;111(16):273–279.
3. Attal N, Cruccu G, Haanpaa M, et al. EFNS guidelines on pharmacological treatment of neuropathic pain. *Eur J Neurol.* 2006;13(11):1153–1169.
4. Bennett M. The LANSS pain scale: the Leeds assessment of neuropathic symptoms and signs. *Pain.* 2001;92(1–2):147–157.

5. Bertelli JA, Ghizoni MF. Pain after avulsion injuries and complete palsy of the brachial plexus: the possible role of nonavulsed roots in pain generation. *Neurosurgery.* 2008;62(5):1104–1113; discussion 1113–1114.
6. Bouhassira D, Attal N, Alchaar H, et al. Comparison of pain syndromes associated with nervous or somatic lesions and development of a new neuropathic pain diagnostic questionnaire (DN4). *Pain.* 2005;114(1–2):29–36.
7. Byrd D, Mackey S. Pulsed radiofrequency for chronic pain. *Curr Pain Headache Rep.* 2008;12(1):37–41.
8. Casscells CD, Lindsey RW, Ebersole J, Li B. Ulnar neuropathy after median sternotomy. *Clin Orthop Relat Res.* 1993;(291):259–265.
9. Cooper DE, Jenkins RS, Bready L, Rockwood CA, Jr. The prevention of injuries of the brachial plexus secondary to malposition of the patient during surgery. *Clin Orthop Relat Res.* 1988;(228):33–41.
10. Deer TR, Skaribas IM, Haider N, et al. Effectiveness of cervical spinal cord stimulation for the management of chronic pain. *Neuromodulation.* 2014;17(3):265–271; discussion 271.
11. Dellon L, Andonian E, Rosson GD. Lower extremity complex regional pain syndrome: long-term outcome after surgical treatment of peripheral pain generators. *J Foot Ankle Surg.* 2010;49(1):33–36.
12. Devor M. The pathophysiology of damaged peripheral nerves. In: Wall PD, Melzack R, eds. *Textbook of Pain.* 3rd ed. Edinburgh: Churchill Livingstone; 1994:79–100.
13. Dworkin RH, O'Connor AB, Audette J, et al. Recommendations for the pharmacological management of neuropathic pain: an overview and literature update. *Mayo Clin Proc.* 2010;85(3 Suppl):S3–S14.
14. Dworkin RH, O'Connor AB, Backonja M, et al. Pharmacologic management of neuropathic pain: evidence-based recommendations. *Pain.* 2007;132(3):237–251.
15. Freynhagen R, Baron R, Gockel U, Tolle TR. painDETECT: a new screening questionnaire to identify neuropathic components in patients with back pain. *Curr Med Res Opin.* 2006;22(10):1911–1920.
16. Gilron I, Watson CP, Cahill CM, Moulin DE. Neuropathic pain: a practical guide for the clinician. *CMAJ.* 2006;175(3):265–275.
17. Goldstein SA, Sturim HS. Intraosseous nerve transposition for treatment of painful neuromas. *J Hand Surg Am.* 1985;10(2):270–274.
18. Gruber H, Glodny B, Kopf H, et al. Practical experience with sonographically guided phenol instillation of stump neuroma: predictors of effects, success, and outcome. *AJR Am J Roentgenol.* 2008;190(5):1263–1269.
19. Haninec P, Kaiser R, Mencl L, Waldauf P. Usefulness of screening tools in the evaluation of long-term effectiveness of DREZ lesioning in the treatment of neuropathic pain after brachial plexus injury. *BMC Neurol.* 2014;14:225.

20. Harden RN, Bruehl S, Perez RS, et al. Validation of proposed diagnostic criteria (the "Budapest Criteria") for Complex Regional Pain Syndrome. *Pain.* 2010;150(2):268–274.

21. Jacob AK, Mantilla CB, Sviggum HP, Schroeder DR, Pagnano MW, Hebl JR. Perioperative nerve injury after total hip arthroplasty: regional anesthesia risk during a 20-year cohort study. *Anesthesiology.* 2011;115(6):1172–1178.

22. Jones RC, 3rd, Lawson E, Backonja M. Managing neuropathic pain. *Med Clin North Am.* 2016;100(1):151–167.

23. Karakaya D, Baris S, Guldogus F, Incesu L, Sarihasan B, Tur A. Brachial plexus injury during subclavian vein catheterization for hemodialysis. *J Clin Anesth.* 2000; 12(3):220–223.

24. Krause SJ, Backonja MM. Development of a neuropathic pain questionnaire. *Clin J Pain.* 2003;19(5):306–314.

25. Kretschmer T, Antoniadis G, Borm W, Richter HP. Iatrogenic nerve injuries. Part 1: frequency distribution, new aspects, and timing of microsurgical treatment. *Chirurg.* 2004;75(11):1104–1112.

26. Kretschmer T, Antoniadis G, Braun V, Rath SA, Richter HP. Evaluation of iatrogenic lesions in 722 surgically treated cases of peripheral nerve trauma. *J Neurosurg.* 2001;94(6):905–912.

27. Kretschmer T, Heinen CW, Antoniadis G, Richter HP, Konig RW. Iatrogenic nerve injuries. In: Spinner RJ, Winfree CJ, eds. *Neurosurgery Clinics of North America. Vol. 20.* Philadelphia, PA: W.B. Saunders Company; 2004:73–90.

28. Laborde KJ, Kalisman M, Tsai TM. Results of surgical treatment of painful neuromas of the hand. *J Hand Surg Am.* 1982;7(2):190–193.

29. Melzack R, Wall PD. Pain mechanisms: a new theory. *Science.* 1965;150(3699):971–979.

30. Navarro X, Vivo M, Valero-Cabre A. Neural plasticity after peripheral nerve injury and regeneration. *Prog Neurobiol.* 2007;82(4):163–201.

31. North RB, Kidd DH, Campbell JN, Long DM. Dorsal root ganglionectomy for failed back surgery syndrome: a 5-year follow-up study. *J Neurosurg.* 1991;74(2):236–242.

32. Novak CB, van Vliet D, Mackinnon SE. Subjective outcome following surgical management of upper extremity neuromas. *J Hand Surg Am.* 1995;20(2):221–226.

33. Novakovic SD, Tzoumaka E, McGivern JG, et al. Distribution of the tetrodotoxin-resistant sodium channel PN3 in rat sensory neurons in normal and neuropathic conditions. *J Neurosci.* 1998;18(6):2174–2187.

34. Osgood CP, Dujovny M, Faille R, Abassy M. Microsurgical lumbosacral ganglionectomy, anatomic rationale, and surgical results. *Acta Neurochir (Wien).* 1976;35(1–3): 197–204.

35. Portenoy R. Development and testing of a neuropathic pain screening questionnaire: ID pain. *Curr Med Res Opin*. 2006;22(8):1555–1565.

36. Staff NP, Engelstad J, Klein CJ, et al. Post-surgical inflammatory neuropathy. *Brain*. 2010;133(10):2866–2880.

37. Stokvis A, van der Avoort DJ, van Neck JW, Hovius SE, Coert JH. Surgical management of neuroma pain: a prospective follow-up study. *Pain*. 2010;151(3):862–869.

38. Thoma A, Veltri K, Haines T, Duku E. A meta-analysis of randomized controlled trials comparing endoscopic and open carpal tunnel decompression. *Plast Reconstr Surg*. 2004;114(5):1137–1146.

39. Toth C, Brady S, Hatfield M. The importance of catastrophizing for successful pharmacological treatment of peripheral neuropathic pain. *J Pain Res*. 2014;7:327–338.

40. Treede RD, Jensen TS, Campbell JN, et al. Neuropathic pain: redefinition and a grading system for clinical and research purposes. *Neurology*. 2008;70(18):1630–1635.

41. van Eijs F, Geurts J, van Kleef M, et al. Predictors of pain relieving response to sympathetic blockade in complex regional pain syndrome type 1. *Anesthesiology*. 2012; 116(1):113–121.

42. Watson JC, Huntoon MA. Neurologic evaluation and management of perioperative nerve injury. *Reg Anesth Pain Med*. 2015;40(5):491–501.

43. Weigel R, Capelle HH, Schmelz M, Krauss JK. Selective thoracic ganglionectomy for the treatment of segmental neuropathic pain. *Eur J Pain*. 2012;16(10):1398–1402.

44. Wilbourn AJ. Iatrogenic nerve injuries. *Neurol Clin*. 1998;16(1):55–82.

45. Wilkinson HA, Chan AS. Sensory ganglionectomy: theory, technical aspects, and clinical experience. *J Neurosurg*. 2001;95(1):61–66.

46. Winfree CJ, Kline DG. Intraoperative positioning nerve injuries. *Surg Neurol*. 2005;63(1):5–18; discussion 18.

47. Woolf CJ, Mannion RJ. Neuropathic pain: aetiology, symptoms, mechanisms, and management. *Lancet*. 1999;353(9168):1959–1964.

48. Yuksel F, Kislaoglu E, Durak N, Ucar C, Karacaoglu E. Prevention of painful neuromas by epineural ligatures, flaps and grafts. *Br J Plast Surg*. 1997;50(3):182–185.

49. Zuo D, Zhou Z, Wang H, et al. Endoscopic versus open carpal tunnel release for idiopathic carpal tunnel syndrome: a meta-analysis of randomized controlled trials. *J Orthop Surg Res*. 2015;10:12.

CHAPTER 3

Postdural Puncture Headache

Joseph E. LaGrew, Carter H. Sigmon, and Steven R. Hanling

In 1898, shortly after the discovery of cocaine's anesthetic properties, "cocainization of spinal cord" was attempted successfully by Doctors Bier and Hildebrandt on themselves and small cohort of patients.[18,63,102] After the procedure, Dr. Beir and others described a debilitating headache (HA) as, "a strong pressure on my skull... [that] recurred as soon as I got up." He found that by lying flat, he and his patients felt "perfectly well" until the symptom remitted on its own 4 to 8 days later. The term postdural puncture headache (PDPH) was not adopted until 70 years later[21,61] but has come to be known as one of the more common adverse effects associated with known dural puncture. Since Dr. Bier's original descriptions over a century ago, studies have provided insight into the incidence, presentation, pathophysiology, risk factors, and prevention and treatments of this adverse effect of dural puncture.

PRESENTATION/INCIDENCE

Commonly used diagnostic criteria for PDPH include an HA that worsens within 15 minutes after sitting or standing and improves within 15 minutes after lying down. The PDPH begins within 6 days after a dural puncture and resolves spontaneously after 1 week or within 48 hours after effective treatment of the spinal fluid leak.[25] The HA is accompanied by at least one of the following symptoms: neck stiffness, tinnitus, hypacusia, photophobia, or nausea.[49] Though the positional component has long been described as one of the essential features of PDPH, there may be a small but significant subset of the population that presents without it. One large retrospective study of 27,064 neuraxial anesthetics found that 8 of 142 patients with accidental dural puncture developed an HA without positional features with four of these patients having both confirmed intracranial hypotension and response to treatment with epidural blood patch (EBP).[59]

In addition, it is important to consider other causes of HA in patients with new onset HA following neuraxial anesthesia as PDPH is a relatively rare phenomenon. Early estimates placed the incidence of PDPH in parturients status postneuraxial analgesia between 0.5% and 1.5%[25,97] and a more recent retrospective study of 237,437 neuraxial anesthetics reported an incidence of 0.69%.[32] Incidence is estimated at 1.4% for known dural puncture and is as high as 51% for accidental dural puncture during epidural placement.[32,68] It is important to note that these numbers may be higher than the risk to the general population as these cohorts were composed exclusively of parturients who are at increased risk for PDPH (see Risk Factors below). In contrast to diagnosis of PDPH, other pathology represents the majority of new onset HAs in patients following known dural puncture. Two small retrospective studies estimated the incidence of PDPH amongst all patients with new onset of HA following neuraxial anesthesia to be 16% to 29%.[44,86] Differential diagnosis for HA after dural puncture includes, but is not limited to a variety of benign HAs, infection, medications, intracranial hemorrhage, cerebral venous thrombosis, stroke, and brain tumor (Table 3-1).

Though there may be variants, such as a subset of patients without a positional feature, the commonly accepted definition is a positional HA which begins within 6 days of a dural puncture. The reported incidence varies and the largest cohort studied may represent a subset of the population at increased risk, but PDPH is estimated to result in 0.69% of all neuraxial anesthetics.

TABLE 3-1 **Differential Diagnosis of Headache After Known or Suspected Dural Puncture, Including Considerations for the Parturient**

Differential Diagnosis of Headache After Dural Puncture
Tension headache
Migraine
Caffeine withdrawal headache
Sinus headache
Pre-eclampsia
Postdural puncture headache
Cervicogenic headache
Illicit drugs (cocaine, amphetamines)
Meningitis
Pneumocephalus
Subdural hematoma
Subarachnoid hematoma
Brain tumor
Stroke
Posterior leukoencephalopathy

PATHOPHYSIOLOGY

Dr. Beir and colleagues originally attributed PDPH to a combination of circulatory disturbances and the loss of cerebrospinal fluid[18,102] based on the symptoms the endured while experimenting upon each other with spinal anesthesia. Because he noted a large amount of cerebrospinal fluid was lost in the performance of these early attempts at neuraxial analgesia and the development of postural related HAs were temporally associated with the performance of the procedure, cerebrospinal fluid loss through a puncture of the meninges became the working theory as to why patients experience PDPHs.

Although CSF is constantly produced, a sudden loss in volume could result in meningeal and vascular traction in the cranial vault when a patient is standing. This traction-related pain is thought to decrease when a patient is in a prone position and has been demonstrated with Magnetic Resonance Imaging (MRI) in 1999.[48] Moreover, the sudden positional HA may be linked to a reflexive vasodilatation of cerebral vasculature to maintain a constant cerebral perfusion pressure in the face of decreasing ICP.[45] Finally, it has been postulated that sensitivity to substance P and subsequent upregulation of neurokinin 1 receptors may play a role in PDPH,[17,26] though research validating this finding is lacking.

RISK FACTORS

Gender, age, and history of chronic HA or previous PDPH are all non-modifiable risk factors for the development of a PDPH. Nonparturient females carry an estimated two-fold higher risk for PDPH than male counterparts.[17,96,101] Incidence correlates well with age. Adults in the third decade of life have been shown to be at highest risk of PDPH with significant decline each decade thereafter until the seventh decade of life.[40,58,96,98,99] Pediatric data are significantly less robust, but most have found children less than 10 years of age rarely suffer PDPH with increasing incidence approaching that of adulthood in those aged 13 to 18 years.[19,75,100] Difficulty evaluating younger children may lead to underrepresentation of the true incidence of PDPH in this cohort.[81] Prior history of chronic HA and previous PDPH have been shown to correlate to two to three times greater likelihood of PDPH.[7,26,56] Correlations between BMI and risk of PDPH have shown mixed results with one large study demonstrating a protective effect of obesity (risk reduction for BMI >30 of 14%, 95% CI 5–23, $p = 0.002$)[68] while another found no difference in incidence based on BMI.[64] Race and pregnancy were investigated as well but not found to correlate with increased incidence of PDPH.[17,58]

There are also numerous modifiable risk factors including mode of delivery, needle gauge, needle type, and bevel position. Evidence suggests that cesarean delivery decreases the risk of PDPH in cases of accidental dural puncture during epidural placement from rates of 74% to 83% down to 10% to 53%.[8,52,74] A correlation between length of pushing during vaginal delivery and rate of PDPH is indicative of increased pressure leading to increased CSF loss.[8] Needle bore has been shown to significantly affect the risk of PDPH with increasing gauge correlating to decreased incidence of PDPH.[16,95] Studies that compared cutting to pencil point bevels have shown decreased risk with pencil point needles,[10,39,57,90,93] though no studies to date have shown superiority of one type of pencil point needle over another. With cutting needles, vertical bevel position has been shown to be better than horizontal needle for prevention of PDPH.[69] Strupp and colleagues hypothesized that an additional risk to use of pencil point needles is the possibility of catching a strand of arachnoid mater that enters the needle during outflow of CSF and is threaded back through the dura during needle withdrawal. In support of this theory, this group found a decreased incidence of PDPH from 16% to 5% when the stylet was replaced prior to needle withdrawal.[89] While different resistance media showed no difference in the incidence of PDPH,[79] a significantly increased risk of HA was reported with air injection in one large prospective study.[4] This difference persisted for only 24 hours and was likely the result of intrathecal air[43] which results in a nonpositional HA immediately following injection. Use of ultrasound, combined spinal–epidural compared to epidural techniques, number of catheter orifices, operator experience, patient position, and preanesthetic hydration status have also been evaluated with no significant effect on the incidence of PDPH.[50,58,76,77,82]

It is difficult to correlate the relative risk found in most of these studies to absolute numbers as most were taken from cohorts that had dural puncture from spinal anesthesia or diagnostic lumbar puncture. Female gender, age, prior history of chronic HA or PDPH, mode of delivery, needle gauge, needle type, and bevel position all have good evidence to support these variables as risk factors for PDPH.

PROPHYLAXIS

Though prevention of dural puncture may be the best prophylaxis of PDPH, several treatments have been assessed for prevention of HA in the case of known dural puncture.[9,13,20,43] Evidence supporting the use of prophylactic EBP is varied with four of five randomized, controlled trials showing benefit following dural puncture with a 17- or 18-gauge needle[3,29,60,74,84]; however, the only double blinded study to include a sham patch showed no significant reduction in the incidence of PDPH (56% in both intervention and control groups).[74] Given the heterogeneity in the literature to date,[9] this treatment should be considered in patients at high risk for PDPH or for those in whom access to the epidural space was technically challenging.[85]

Medical prophylaxis for PDPH has been shown to be effective, supported by a few small, though well designed, studies.[1,6,33,46,73] Morphine injected into epidural space in 3-mg doses 24 hours apart was shown to be beneficial in reducing incidence of PDPH (RR 0.25, 05% CI 0.08–0.78)[5] though the treatment group had a higher incidence of nausea, vomiting, and pruritus. In addition, a second dose of epidural morphine would extend hospital stay for monitoring of delayed respiratory depression.[43] Spinal opioids, however, have shown no benefit (morphine compared to placebo RR 1.18, 95% CI 0.51–2.76 and fentanyl compared to no intervention RR 1.79, 95% CI 0.54–5.91, respectively).[1,33] IV cosyntropin 1 mg given over 5 minutes following vaginal delivery in patients with accidental dural puncture was demonstrated to reduce the risk of PDPH (RR 0.49, 95% CI 0.31–0.79)[46] and 1 to 1.5 mg/kg of IV aminophylline given after cord clamping was shown to decrease the rate of PDPH following spinal anesthesia for caesarian section (RR 0.16, CI 95% 0.05–0.51).[73] The later study evaluated dural puncture after spinal anesthesia with a smaller gauge needle and did not describe side effects of the treatment and control groups. Other drugs including intravenous caffeine, intravenous dexamethasone, rectal indomethacin, and epidural and intrathecal normal saline have shown no significant benefit in reducing incidence of PDPH.[24,31,34,37,40,87,92,94,103] Tazeh-kand and colleagues demonstrated reduced duration of PDPH (2% persistence of PDPH in the treatment versus 24% in the control group at 3 to 7 days, $p = 0.002$) following 5 mL of intrathecal normal saline injected prior to dosing of the spinal though this was not adjusted for patients receiving EBP as treatment.

Finally, it has been postulated that placement of an intrathecal catheter at the time of an accidental dural puncture, would stimulate fibrosis and result in a smaller dural insult.[12] Pooled analysis of short term catheter placement (removal less than 24 hours after dural puncture) showed no benefit, though evidence is limited to nonrandomized studies and retrospective chart reviews.[9,12,27,65,67,72] Ayad and investigators found a profound difference in catheters left for greater than 24 hours (6.2% vs. 91.9% incidence in the study and control groups); however, a similar sized randomized controlled trial found no decrease in PDPH with intrathecal catheter for greater than 24 hours.[71] Though data on intrathecal catheter placement may be conflicting, the study by Russell and colleagues demonstrated a second accidental dural puncture in one third of patients randomized to receive epidural at another level following dural puncture,[71] suggesting a benefit of prevention of further comorbidities by placing an intrathecal catheter.

The best evidence for pharmacologic prevention of PDPH supports epidural morphine and IV cosyntropin for accidental dural puncture with 16- to 18-gauge Touhy and for aminophylline following puncture with 23- to 25-gauge needles, though evidence is restricted to single, small randomized controlled studies. Studies evaluating prophylactic EBP and placement of intrathecal catheter for at least 24 hours have demonstrated mixed results, but evidence supports a role for these treatments in select patients.

TREATMENTS

PDPHs are typically mild, and most resolve spontaneously. As such, conservative therapy during the initial course is recommended. Conservative therapy includes oral and IV medication, abdominal binders, hydration, and bed rest. Evidence for these modalities is limited to small studies.[11,13,14] Gabapentin 900 mg three times daily has been shown to significantly improve pain scores at 1 to 4 days postpresentation compared to placebo[35] and 300 mg three times daily compared to Ergotamine plus caffeine.[36] Results were similar between the two studies though the cohorts were small and proportion of patients with PDPH was not evaluated in either study. Similarly, hydrocortisone demonstrated improvement compared to placebo[66] and conservative therapy[6] with repeated dosing intravenously for the first 48 hours after onset of PDPH. In addition to limits in study size and outcomes, these studies were also limited by length of follow-up. Theophylline showed a benefit in reduction of average pain scores after a single dose compared to conservative treatment[80] and one day of repeated doses compared to acetaminophen[62] but included no observations beyond 24 hours after treatment. Feuerstein and Zeides[38] showed decreased average pain scores in a very small (n = 11) group treated with theophylline compared to placebo; however, 5 of 16 individuals were unable to complete the study protocol with a bias in this group toward treatment failure. Caffeine has demonstrated benefit compared to placebo in average pain score as well as decrease in proportion of participants with PDPH.[23,78] Intravenous cosyntropin, a synthetic analogue of ACTH, has shown equivalence in efficacy to caffeine[104] and EBP[47] when evaluated primarily in patients with PDPH following diagnostic lumbar puncture. The former study is limited by a short duration of follow-up and was underpowered to detect type II error, and the later study showed equivalence of treatments over 7 days but demonstrated a bimodal response with superiority of EBP at 1 day posttreatment. It should also be noted that one smaller study of intramuscular ACTH compared to placebo showed no benefit in average pain scores.[70] Simvastatin showed marginal improvement[30] and pregabalin showed no benefit[51] compared to placebo. Other modalities, including hydration, bed rest, and abdominal binders have all been recommended, but evidence for their use is limited.[11,95] The majority of studies noted above, looked at patients receiving spinal anesthesia compared to those with diagnostic lumbar puncture or accidental dural puncture during epidural placement and parturients were underrepresented in these studies.

PDPHs that have not responded to conservative measures, or are severe in nature, may benefit from more invasive procedures. EBP is currently the standard treatment for severe PDPH or for mild cases refractory to conservative measures.[13] EBP was originally thought to be 90% effective with repeat treatment efficacy approaching >96%; however, studies with increased patient follow up showed persistent relief of symptoms in 61% to 75% of treatments.[22,88,91] Treatment with EBP requires trained personnel to perform,[41] has numerous contraindications and has been associated with rare but serious complications to include severe back pain, bradycardia, neurologic deterioration, postpartum seizures, and cranial nerve paresis.[2,3,15,42,,83,88]

More recently, sphenopalatine ganglion block (SPGB) has been suggested as less invasive alternative to EBP for treating PDPH. SPGBs have traditionally been used to treat causes of head and facial pain including migraines, cluster HAs and trigeminal neuralgia.[54,55] The SPGB can be performed via a transnasal approach with cotton-tip applicators soaked in local anesthetic solution, viscous lidocaine or several catheter and syringes kits purpose built for in office sphenopalatine injections.[53] It can be repeated once a day for a week, and in one institution, performed by the patient at home with proper instruction. In a small case series, 69% of patients were saved from having to undergo an EBP.[28] Compared with EBP, SPGBs offer improved safety, may be more cost-effective, and are less invasive to the patient.[28] Further research with increased sample size and longer follow up are needed to more clearly delineate the efficacy of this emerging treatment.

In summary, treatment of PDPH is directed first at medical treatment options with good evidence, limited by smaller studies, supporting caffeine, gabapentin, cosyntropin, and hydrocortisone with EBP reserved for severe or refractory HA. SPGB has shown promise as a less invasive option, but further studies are needed to elucidate its role in treatment of PDPH.

REFERENCES

1. Abboud TK, Zhu J, Reyes A, et al. Effect of subarachnoid morphine on the incidence of spinal headache. *Reg Anesth.* 1992;17(1):34–36.
2. Abouleish E, Vega S, Blendinger I, Tio TO. Long-term follow-up of epidural blood patch. *Anesth Analg.* 1975;54(4):459–463.
3. Ackerman WE, Juneja MM, Kaczorowski DM. Prophylactic epidural blood patch for the prevention of postdural puncture headache in the parturient. *Anesthesiol Rev.* 1990;17:45–49.
4. Aida S, Taga K, Yamakura T, Endoh H, Shimoji K. Headache after attempted epidural block the role of intrathecal air. *Anesthesiology.* 1998;88(1):76–81.
5. Al-metwalli RR. Epidural morphine injections for prevention of post dural puncture headache. *Anaesthesia.* 2008;63(8):847–850.
6. Alam MR, Rahman MA, Ershad R. Role of very short-term intravenous hydrocortisone in reducing postdural puncture headache. *J Anaesthesiol Clin Pharmacol.* 2012; 28(2):190–193.

7. Amorim JA, Valença MM. Postdural puncture headache is a risk factor for new post-dural puncture headache. *Cephalalgia.* 2008;28(1):5–8.
8. Angle P, Thompson D, Halpern S, Wilson DB. Second stage pushing correlates with headache after unintentional dural puncture in parturients. *Can J Anaesth.* 1999;46(9):861–866.
9. Apfel CC, Saxena A, Cakmakkaya OS, Gaiser R, George E, Radke O. Prevention of postdural puncture headache after accidental dural puncture: a quantitative systematic review. *Br J Anaesth.* 2010;105(3):255–263.
10. Apiliogullari S, Duman A, Gok F, Akillioglu I. Spinal needle design and size affect the incidence of postdural puncture headache in children. *Paediatr Anaesth.* 2010; 20(2):177–182.
11. Arevalo-Rodriguez I, Ciapponi A, Munoz L, Roque i Figuls M, Bonfill Cosp X. Posture and fluids for preventing post-dural puncture headache. *Cochrane Database Syst Rev.* 2013;(7):CD009199.
12. Ayad S, Demian Y, Narouze SN, Tetzlaff JE. Subarachnoid catheter placement after wet tap for analgesia in labor: influence on the risk of headache in obstetric patients. *Reg Anesth Pain Med.* 2003;28(6):512–515.
13. Basurto Ona X, Martínez García L, Solà I, Bonfill Cosp X. Drug therapy for treating post-dural puncture headache. *Cochrane Database Syst Rev.* 2011;(8):CD007887.
14. Basurto Ona X, Osorio D, Bonfill Cosp X. Drug therapy for treating post-dural puncture headache. *Cochrane Database Syst Rev.* 2015;(7):CD007887.
15. Beers RA, Cambareri JJ, Rodziewicz GS. Acute deterioration of mental status follow ing epidural blood patch. *Anesth Analg.* 1993;76(5):1147–1149.
16. Bezov D, Ashina S, Lipton R. Post-dural puncture headache: part II–prevention, management, and prognosis. *Headache.* 2010;50(9):1482–1498.
17. Bezov D, Lipton RB, Ashina S. Post-dural puncture headache: part I diagnosis, epidemiology, etiology, and pathophysiology. *Headache.* 2010;50(7):1144–1152.
18. Bier A. Versuche über cocainisirung des rückenmarkes. *Deutsche Zeitschrift für Chirurgie.* 1899;51(3–4):361–369.
19. Bolder PM. Postlumbar puncture headache in pediatric oncology patients. *Anesthesiology.* 1986;65(6):696–698.
20. Bradbury CL, Singh SI, Badder SR, Wakely LJ, Jones PM. Prevention of post-dural puncture headache in parturients: a systematic review and meta-analysis. *Acta Anaesthesiol Scand.* 2013;57(4):417–430.
21. Bridenbaugh PO. Postdural puncture headache. *Reg Anesth Pain Med.* 1978;3(1):5–6.
22. Brownridge P. The management of headache following accidental dural puncture in obstetric patients. *Anaesth Intensive Care.* 1983;11(1):4–15.

23. Camann WR, Murray RS, Mushlin PS, Lambert DH. Effects of oral caffeine on postdural puncture headache. A double-blind, placebo-controlled trial. *Anesth Analg.* 1990;70(2):181–184.

24. Charsley MM, Abram SE. The injection of intrathecal normal saline reduces the severity of postdural puncture headache. *Reg Anesth Pain Med.* 2001;26(4): 301–305.

25. Choi PT, Galinski SE, Takeuchi L, Lucas S, Tamayo C, Jadad AR. PDPH is a common complication of neuraxial blockade in parturients: a meta-analysis of obstetrical studies. *Can J Anesth.* 2003;50(5):460–469.

26. Clark JW, Solomon GD, Senanayake PD, Gallagher C. Substance P concentration and history of headache in relation to postlumbar puncture headache: towards prevention. *J Neurol Neurosurg Psychiatry.* 1996;60(6):681–683.

27. Cohen S, Amar D, Pantuck EJ, Singer N, Divon M. Decreased incidence of headache after accidental dural puncture in caesarean delivery patients receiving continuous postoperative intrathecal analgesia. *Acta Anaesthesiol Scand.* 1994;38(7):716–718.

28. Cohen S, Ramos D, Grubb W, Mellender S, Mohiuddin A, Chiricolo A. Sphenopalatine ganglion block: a safer alternative to epidural blood patch for postdural puncture headache. *Reg Anesth Pain Med.* 2014;39(6):563.

29. Colonna-Romano P, Shapiro BE. Unintentional dural puncture and prophylactic epidural blood patch in obstetrics. *Anesth Analg.* 1989;69(4):522–523.

30. Connelly NR, Parker RK, Rahimi A, Gibson CS. Sumatriptan in patients with postdural puncture headache. *Headache.* 2000;40(4):316–319.

31. Craft JB, Epstein BS, Coakley CS. Prophylaxis of dural-puncture headache with epidural saline. *Anesth Analg.* 1973;52(2):228–231.

32. D'Angelo R, Smiley RM, Riley ET, Segal S. Serious complications related to obstetric anesthesia: the serious complication repository project of the society for obstetric anesthesia and perinatology. *Anesthesiology.* 2014;120(6):1505–1512.

33. Devcic A, Sprung J, Patel S, Kettler R, Maitra-D'cruze A. PDPH in obstetric anesthesia: Comparison of 24-gauge sprotte and 25-gauge quincke needles and effect of subarachnoid administration of fentanyl. *Reg Anesth.* 1993;18(4):222–225.

34. Doroudian MR, Norouzi M, Esmailie M, Tanhaeivash R. Dexamethasone in preventing post-dural puncture headache: a randomized, double-blind, placebo-controlled trial. *Acta Anaesthesiol Belg.* 2011;62(3):143–146.

35. Erol DD. The effect of oral gabapentin on postdural puncture headache. *Acute Pain.* 2006;8(4):169–173.

36. Erol DD. The analgesic and antiemetic efficacy of gabapentin or ergotamine/caffeine for the treatment of postdural puncture headache. *Adv Med Sci.* 2011;56(1):25–29.

37. Esmaoglu A, Akpinar H, Uğur F. Oral multidose caffeine-paracetamol combination is not effective for the prophylaxis of postdural puncture headache. *J Clin Anesth.* 2005;17(1):58–61.

38. Feuerstein TJ, Zeides A. Theophylline relieves headache following lumbar puncture. Placebo-controlled, double-blind pilot study. *Klin Wochenschr.* 1986;64(5):216–218.

39. Flaatten H, Felthaus J, Kuwelker M, Wisborg T. Postural post-dural puncture headache. A prospective randomised study and a meta-analysis comparing two different 0.40 mm OD (27 g) spinal needles. *Acta Anaesthesiol Scand.* 2000;44(6):643–647.

40. Flaatten H, Rodt S, Rosland J, Vamnes J. Postoperative headache in young patients after spinal anaesthesia. *Anaesthesia.* 1987;42(2):202–205.

41. Frank RL. Lumbar puncture and post-dural puncture headaches: implications for the emergency physician. *J Emerg Med.* 2008;35(2):149–157.

42. Frison LM, Dorsey DL. Epidural blood patch and late postpartum eclampsia. *Anesth Analg.* 1996;82(3):666–668.

43. Gaiser RR. Postdural puncture headache: an evidence-based approach. *Anesthesiol Clin.* 2017;35(1):157–167.

44. Goldszmidt E, Kern R, Chaput A, Macarthur A. The incidence and etiology of postpartum headaches: a prospective cohort study. *Can J Anaesth.* 2005;52(9):971–977.

45. Grant R, Condon B, Hart I, Teasdale GM. Changes in intracranial CSF volume after lumbar puncture and their relationship to post-LP headache. *J Neurol Neurosurg Psychiatry.* 1991;54(5):440–442.

46. Hakim SM. Cosyntropin for prophylaxis against postdural puncture headache after accidental dural puncture. *Anesthesiology.* 2010;113(2):413–420.

47. Hanling SR, Lagrew JE, 2nd, Colmenar DH, Quiko AS, Drastol CA. Intravenous cosyntropin versus epidural blood patch for treatment of postdural puncture headache. *Pain Med.* 2016;17(7):1337–1342.

48. Hannerz J, Ericson K, Bro Skejø HP. MR imaging with gadolinium in patients with and without post-lumbar puncture headache. *Acta Radiol.* 1999;40(2):135–141.

49. Headache Classification Committee of the International Headache Society (IHS). The international classification of headache disorders, 3rd edition (beta version). *Cephalalgia.* 2013;33(9):629–808.

50. Heesen M, Klohr S, Rossaint R, Van De Velde M, Straube S. Can the incidence of accidental dural puncture in laboring women be reduced? A systematic review and meta-analysis. *Minerva Anestesiol.* 2013;79(10):1187–1197.

51. Huseyinoglu U, Huseyinoglu N, Hamurtekin E, Aygun H, Sulu B. Effect of pregabalin on post-dural-puncture headache following spinal anesthesia and lumbar puncture. *J Clin Neurosci.* 2011;18(10):1365–1368.

52. Jagannathan DK, Arriaga AF, Elterman KG, et al. Effect of neuraxial technique after inadvertent dural puncture on obstetric outcomes and anesthetic complications. *Int J Obstet Anesth*. 2016;25:23–29.

53. Katz D, Beilin Y. Review of the alternatives to epidural blood patch for treatment of postdural puncture headache in the parturient. *Anesth Analg*. 2017;124(4):1219–1228.

54. Kent S, Mehaffey G. Transnasal sphenopalatine ganglion block for the treatment of postdural puncture headache in the ED. *Am J Emerg Med*. 2015;33(11):1714.e1–e2.

55. Kent S, Mehaffey G. Transnasal sphenopalatine ganglion block for the treatment of postdural puncture headache in obstetric patients. *J Clin Anesth*. 2016;34:194–196.

56. Kuntz KM, Kokmen E, Stevens JC, Miller P, Offord KP, Ho MM. Post-lumbar puncture headaches: experience in 501 consecutive procedures. *Neurology*. 1992; 42(10):1884–1887.

57. Lavi R, Yarnitsky D, Rowe JM, Weissman A, Segal D, Avivi I. Standard vs atraumatic whitacre needle for diagnostic lumbar puncture: a randomized trial. *Neurology*. 2006; 67(8):1492–1494.

58. Leibold RA, Yealy DM, Coppola M, Cantees KK. Post-dural-puncture headache: characteristics, management, and prevention. *Ann Emerg Med*. 1993;22(12):1863–1870.

59. Loures V, Savoldelli G, Kern K, Haller G. Atypical headache following dural puncture in obstetrics. *Int J Obstet Anesth*. 2014;23(3):246–252.

60. Lowenwirt I, Cohen S, Zephyr J, Hamer R, Hronkova B, Rovner JS. Can prophylactic epidural blood patch reduce the incidence and severity of postpartum dural puncture headache in obstetrics? *Anesth Analg*. 1998;86(2S):378S.

61. Lund PC. *Principles and Practice of Spinal Anesthesia*. Sprinfield, IL: Charles T. Thomas; 1971.

62. Mahoori A, Hassani E, Noroozinia H, Javaheri N, Hatami S. Theophylline versus acetaminophen in the treatment of post-dural puncture headache (PDPH). *Middle East J Anaesthesiol*. 2013;22(3):289–292.

63. Marx GF. The first spinal anesthesia. Who deserves the laurels? *Reg Anesth*. 1994;19(6):429–430.

64. Miu M, Paech MJ, Nathan E. The relationship between body mass index and post-dural puncture headache in obstetric patients. *In J Obstet Anesth*. 2014;23(4): 371–375.

65. Norris MC, Leighton BL. Continuous spinal anesthesia after unintentional dural puncture in parturients. *Reg Anesth*. 1990;15(6):285–287.

66. Noyan Ashraf MA, Sadeghi A, Azarbakht Z, Salehi S, Hamediseresht E. Evaluation of intravenous hydrocortisone in reducing headache after spinal anesthesia:

a double blind controlled clinical study [corrected]. *Middle East J Anaesthesiol.* 2007;19(2):415–422.

67. Paech M, Banks S, Gurrin L. An audit of accidental dural puncture during epidural insertion of a tuohy needle in obstetric patients. *Int J Obstet Anesth.* 2001;10(3): 162–167.

68. Peralta F, Higgins N, Lange E, Wong CA, McCarthy RJ. The relationship of body mass index with the incidence of postdural puncture headache in parturients. *Anesth Analg.* 2015;121(2):451–456.

69. Richman JM, Joe EM, Cohen SR, et al. Bevel direction and postdural puncture headache: a meta-analysis. *Neurologist.* 2006;12(4):224–228.

70. Rucklidge MW, Yentis SM, Paech MJ. Synacthen depot for the treatment of postdural puncture headache. *Anaesthesia.* 2004;59(2):138–141.

71. Russell IF. A prospective controlled study of continuous spinal analgesia versus repeat epidural analgesia after accidental dural puncture in labour. *Int J Obstet Anesth.* 2012;21(1):7–16.

72. Rutter SV, Shields F, Broadbent CR, Popat M, Russell R. Management of accidental dural puncture in labour with intrathecal catheters: an analysis of 10 years' experience. *Int J Obstet Anesth.* 2001;10(3):177–181.

73. Sadeghi SE, Abdollahifard G, Nasabi NA, Mehrabi M, Safarpour AR. Effectiveness of single dose intravenous aminophylline administration on prevention of post dural puncture headache in patients who received spinal anesthesia for elective cesarean section. *World J Med Sci.* 2012;7(1):13–16.

74. Scavone BM, Wong CA, Sullivan JT, Yaghmour E, Sherwani SS, McCarthy RJ. Efficacy of a prophylactic epidural blood patch in preventing post dural puncture headache in parturients after inadvertent dural puncture. *Anesthesiology.* 2004;101(6):1422–1427.

75. Scher C, Ginsburg I, Amar D, Rensil R, McDowall R, Barst S. Post dural puncture headache in children with cancer. *Reg Anesth Pain Med.* 1992;17(3):91.

76. Schier R, Guerra D, Aguilar J, et al. Epidural space identification: a meta-analysis of complications after air versus liquid as the medium for loss of resistance. *Anesth Analg.* 2009;109(6):2012–2021.

77. Schnabel A, Schuster F, Ermert T, Eberhart LH, Metterlein T, Kranke P. Ultrasound guidance for neuraxial analgesia and anesthesia in obstetrics: a quantitative systematic review. *Ultraschall Med.* 2012;33(7):E132–E137.

78. Sechzer PH. Post-spinal anesthesia headache treated with caffeine. Part II: intracranial vascular distension. A key factor. *Survey Anesthesiol.* 1981;25(1):55–56.

79. Segal S, Arendt KW. A retrospective effectiveness study of loss of resistance to air or saline for identification of the epidural space. *Anesth Analg.* 2010;110(2):558–563.

80. Sen J, Sen B. Non invasive management of post dural puncture headache-A comparison. *BJMS*. 2014;13(2):114.

81. Sethna NF, Berde CB. Pediatric regional anesthesia. *Pediatr Anesth*. 1994;1:647–678.

82. Simmons SW, Taghizadeh N, Dennis AT, Hughes D, Cyna AM. Combined spinal-epidural versus epidural analgesia in labour. *Cochrane Database Syst Rev*. 2012;10: CD003401.

83. Sperry RJ, Gartrell A, Johnson JO. Epidural blood patch can cause acute neurologic deterioration. *Anesthesiology*. 1995;82(1):303–305.

84. Stein MH, Cohen S, Mohiuddin MA, Dombrovskiy V, Lowenwirt I. Prophylactic vs therapeutic blood patch for obstetric patients with accidental dural puncture–a randomised controlled trial. *Anaesthesia*. 2014;69(4):320–326.

85. Stein MH, Cohen S, Mohiuddin MA, Dombrovskiy V, Lowenwirt I. Prophylactic versus therapeutic blood patch for obstetric patients with accidental dural puncture: a randomized controlled trial. *Obstetric Anesthesia Digest*. 2015;35(1):28–29.

86. Stella CL, Jodicke CD, How HY, Harkness UF, Sibai BM. Postpartum headache: is your work-up complete?. *Am J Obstet Gynecol*. 2007;196(4):318.e1–e7.

87. Strelec S, Prylinski J, Sakert T, Royal M. The efficacy of multi-dose oral caffeine in prevention of post-dural puncture headache. *Reg Anesth Pain Med*. 1994; 19(2):79.

88. Stride PC, Cooper GM. Dural taps revisited. A 20-year survey from Birmingham Maternity Hospital. *Anaesthesia*. 1993;48(3):247–255.

89. Strupp M, Brandt T, Müller A. Incidence of post-lumbar puncture syndrome reduced by reinserting the stylet: a randomized prospective study of 600 patients. *J Neurol*. 1998;245(9):589–592.

90. Strupp M, Schueler O, Straube A, Von Stuckrad-Barre S, Brandt T. "Atraumatic" sprotte needle reduces the incidence of post-lumbar puncture headaches. *Neurology*. 2001;57(12):2310–2312.

91. Taivainen T, Pitkänen M, Tuominen M, Rosenberg PH. Efficacy of epidural blood patch for postdural puncture headache. *Acta Anaesthesiol Scand*. 1993;37(7):702–705.

92. Tazeh-kand NF, Eslami B, Marzony SG, Abolhassani R, Mohammadian K. Injection of intrathecal normal saline in decreasing postdural puncture headache. *J Anesth*. 2014;28(2):206–209.

93. Thomas SR, Jamieson DR, Muir KW. Randomised controlled trial of atraumatic versus standard needles for diagnostic lumbar puncture. *BMJ*. 2000;321(7267):986–990.

94. Trivedi NS, Eddi D, Shevde K. Headache prevention following accidental dural puncture in obstetric patients. *J Clin Anesth*. 1993;5(1):42–45.

95. Turnbull DK, Shepherd DB. Post-dural puncture headache: pathogenesis, prevention and treatment. *Br J Anaesth*. 2003;91(5):718–729.

96. Vandam LD, Dripps RD. Long-term follow-up of patients who received 10,098 spinal anesthetics: syndrome of decreased intracranial pressure (headache and ocular and auditory difficulties). *J Am Med Assoc*. 1956;161(7):586–591.

97. Van De Velde M, Teunkens A, Hanssens M, Van Assche FA, Vandermeersch E. Post dural puncture headache following combined spinal epidural or epidural anaesthesia in obstetric patients. *Anaesth Intensive Care*. 2001;29(6):595.

98. Vilming ST, Kloster R. Post-lumbar puncture headache: clinical features and suggestions for diagnostic criteria. *Cephalalgia*. 1997;17(7):778–784.

99. Wadud R, Laiq N, Qureshi FA, Jan AS. The frequency of postdural puncture headache in different age groups. *J Coll Physicians Surg Pak*. 2006;16(6):389–392.

100. Wee LH, Lam F, Cranston AJ. The incidence of post dural puncture headache in children. *Anaesthesia*. 1996;51(12):1164–1166.

101. Wu CL, Rowlingson AJ, Cohen SR, et al. Gender and post-dural puncture headache. *Anesthesiology*. 2006;105(3):613–618.

102. Wulf HF. The centennial of spinal anesthesia. *Anesthesiology*. 1998;89(2):500–506.

103. Yousefshahi F, Dahmardeh AR, Khajavi M, Najafi A, Khashayar P, Barkhordari K. Effect of dexamethasone on the frequency of postdural puncture headache after spinal anesthesia for cesarean section: a double-blind randomized clinical trial. *Acta Neurol Belg*. 2012;112(4):345–350.

104. Zeger W, Younggren B, Smith L. Comparison of cosyntropin versus caffeine for post-dural puncture headaches: a randomized double-blind trial. *World J Emerg Med*. 2012;3(3):182–185.

CHAPTER 4

Pain from Gastrointestinal Surgery

Asbjørn Mohr Drewes

Communication from the viscera does not normally reach consciousness, except for information due to filling of the esophagus, stomach, and rectum. On the other hand, when the organs are potentially in danger, for example, due to surgery or diseases, symptoms such as discomfort and pain are sensed. These symptoms are typically vague and difficult to characterize, and are often quite distinct from what is felt after noxious stimuli of the somatic system. The anatomical structure and organization of the visceral nervous systems explains to a major degree the symptoms experienced after abdominal surgery. This has been discovered in more detail over the last decades. Most of our basic knowledge about visceral pain processing in the nervous system is taken from animal experiments. However, there are major differences between species in the organization of the pain system and preclinical data after surgery can be difficult to interpret. Recently, there has been an increasing knowledge about visceral pain from human studies, and translational findings, experimental and clinical research has increased and supplement each other. This chapter gives a short introduction to the visceral pain system followed by an explanation of the rationale for experimental pain models in these settings, and finally a section about pain following abdominal surgery.

THE VISCERAL PAIN SYSTEM

In the following section, the visceral pain system is briefly described to facilitate the understanding of the clinical symptoms that may arise after surgery.

The viscera have a complex dual innervation with both intrinsic and extrinsic sensory neurons (visceral afferents). The innervation pattern may, to some degree, explain the clinical characteristics of visceral pain that is typically diffuse and unpleasant, and associated with referred pain to somatic structures as well as autonomic symptoms such as sweating and nausea (Fig. 4-1). Intrinsic afferents project locally in the wall of the gut and are involved in regulation of physiologic functions, such as secretion, motility, mucosal transport, and blood flow.[16] Extrinsic afferents project to the central nervous system (CNS) either (a) via the vagal nerve to the brain stem or (b) through splanchnic nerves to the spinal cord (Table 4-1).[48] The vagal afferents are believed mainly to mediate nonnoxious physiologic sensations such as satiety and nausea (low-response thresholds).[2] However, vagal afferents may also be involved in the central inhibitory modulation of pain.[45] In case

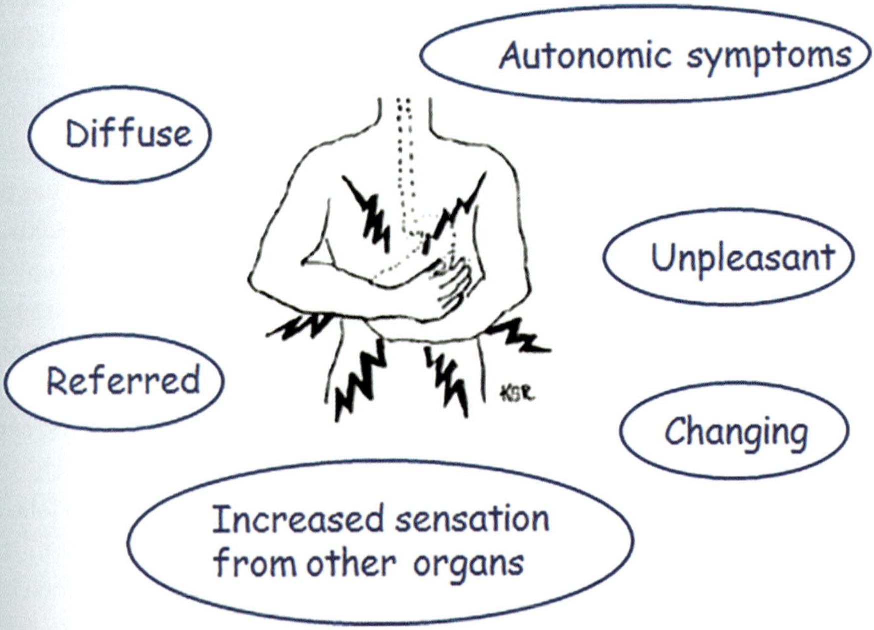

FIGURE 4-1 Characteristics of visceral pain.

TABLE 4-1 General Characteristics of Pain Due to Visceral Pathology
1. Is poorly localized with referral to somatic structures
2. Produces nonspecific regional or whole-body motor responses
3. Produces strong autonomic responses
4. Leads to sensitization of somatic tissues
5. Produces strong affective responses

of transmural inflammation after surgery, the peritoneum may be affected, and as this has somatic-like fibers the appearance of pain is changed to a distinct and well-characterized pain pattern (Table 4-1).

Normally visceral pain is conveyed to the spinal cord, where the afferents run in parallel with the sympathetic fibers. The afferent projections are organized in a somewhat segmental manner, but distributed over several spinal segments in both rostral and caudal directions (Table 4-1).[31] The diffuse spinal termination pattern may explain the poor localization of visceral sensations often seen in clinical practice such as after surgery.[15] From the spinal cord, pain transmits to the brain through diverse pathways. Most afferents travel in the spinothalamic tract to the thalamus. From the thalamus, there are projections to the insula, hypothalamus, amygdala, as well as to higher cortical levels such as cingulate and prefrontal cortices. Insula has an important function for integrating the visceral sensory and motor activity and is particularly important in pain perception from the gut.[36] The anterior cingulate cortices and prefrontal cortices are a part of the "medial pain system," which mediates the affective, emotional, and cognitive components of pain experience.[57] In addition to the spinothalamic tract, some afferents ascend in the spinoreticular tract mediating arousal and autonomic responses through interaction with the reticular formation. Finally, a population of afferents ascends in the spinomesencephalic tract, which relates to a complex neuronal network including the periaqueductal gray, rostroventral medulla and the dorsolateral pontine tegmentum. This network comprises the structural basis of descending pain control and possesses modulation of spinal pain processing.[29]

As each segment in the spinal cord receives afferent fibers from visceral as well as somatic structures, visceral pain is often reported in a somatic area (*referred pain*). Although simplified, referred pain originates due to convergence between visceral and somatic fibers on the same second-order neuron (for details, see Arendt-Nielsen et al.[3] and Qin et al.[44]). Since the brain cannot localize the precise origin of the visceral pain stimulus, it may therefore interpret the pain as originating from a somatic structure with the same segmental innervation. Pain can also manifest in neighbor organs that are not affected by disease or surgery. *Viscero-visceral hyperalgesia* is a complex form of hypersensitivity probably explained by more than one mechanism. Since this phenomenon takes place between visceral organs sharing their central afferent terminations, it is plausible that central sensitization plays an important role.[23] For example, our group has shown that esophageal perfusion with acid and capsaicin increased the sensitivity in the rectum.[13,46] Besides changes at the spinal level, changes in the cortical processing of pain may be involved in these mechanisms.[24] Viscero-visceral hyperalgesia may explain the epidemiologic findings that several clinical conditions with organic diseases show evidence of increased pain from other organs. This was investigated in patients suffering from, among others, coronary artery disease and gallbladder stones, or inflammatory bowel disease and dysmenorrhea.[5] In these studies, coexisting visceral pain conditions with a share of spinal projections between organs increased the symptoms generated from the other pain condition. In addition, effective treatment of one condition significantly improved symptoms from the other. Although not proven in experimental or clinical studies, such affections of remote viscera are often seen after surgery and it is plausible that mechanisms are, to a high degree, similar.

Investigation of Visceral Pain—Experimental Methods

Our knowledge about pain after surgery in humans is, to a major degree, based on clinical studies. However, pain in patients is often blurred and difficult to evaluate due to other symptoms such as medication (especially in the postoperative settings), anxiety, and cognitive consequences of the pain. Furthermore, sedative properties of some analgesics make evaluation difficult. Experimental methods to evoke and assess pain under controlled circumstances are advantageous as they encompass many of these problems and offer a unique opportunity to investigate effects on different pain modalities arising from different tissues as well as peripheral and central pain mechanisms (for details, see Arendt-Nielsen and Yarnitsky[4] and Drewes et al.[18]). Methods to deliver controlled and reliable stimulation of the esophagus, stomach, small intestine, and large intestine are well described and can be both phasic, tonic, and multimodal. In addition, models can evoke allodynia and hyperalgesia and as such mimic clinical pain. Such models reflect symptoms seen after surgery although their simple nature of cause may limit any generalizations.

Several studies have confirmed previous animal experiments, showing that sensitization of the human gut (e.g., acid perfusion of the esophagus) results in CNS alterations reflected in an increase in the referred pain area as well as a lowering of the pain thresholds to stimulation of other organs.[19] Such changes thought to be mainly spinal, may be modality specific and influenced by descending modulation. Hence, in a subsequent study where a more intense sensitization model was used (perfusion of the esophagus with *both* acid and capsaicin), rectal hyperalgesia to heat and mechanical stimulations was observed.[22] The sensitization may also lead to profound changes in the autonomous systems and thereby influence the brain's so-called pain matrix.[13]

The evoked sensations can be assessed with subjective methods quantitatively (e.g., by using a visual analog scale) and qualitatively (e.g., by using the McGill Pain Questionnaire). Objectively, physiologic responses for the pain can also be recorded with, for example, the nociceptive reflex, cerebral evoked potentials, and imaging. The nociceptive reflex investigates mainly *spinal pathways*, which can be modulated by other afferent inputs, spinal neuronal excitability, and activity in descending control systems. In the studies by Bouhassira et al.,[8,9] tonic distension of the stomach and rectum resulted in inhibition of the reflex. On the other hand, in a study where we distended the esophagus, no change in reflex size was present before sensitization was induced.[21] Therefore, the different stimulation sites and experimental situations may explain the discrepancies between the experiments. At the *brain level* most studies have focused on imaging methods as these have many advantages. For example, functional magnetic resonance imaging (fMRI) has an excellent spatial resolution (2 to 5 mm), especially in the more superficial layers. However, as the temporal resolution ranges from a 300-ms theoretical value to a more realistic 1 to 3 seconds, there will invariably be many biases relating to nonspecific activation and activation of centers and networks not related directly to pain. Neuroimaging has also been based on tools such as positron emission tomography (PET) and magnetoencephalography. Results of these studies are, despite some emerging consistencies, fairly heterogeneous. For a more comprehensive overview, the reader is referred to studies of Sharma et al.[49] and Oudenhove.[41] Although electroencephalography (EEG) methods also have many limitations—some of them shared with fMRI—they are generally highly available, relatively easy to use, and of low cost.[47] The main advantage is the high temporal resolution, which allows assessment of the primary pain processing, including sequential activation and analysis of coherence and cross-talk between brain centers. However, EEG has a relatively poor spatial resolution even though various inverse modeling algorithms and signal decomposition procedures have overcome this limitation to some extent. The results from experimental stimulation of the viscera may, to a large extent, be used to understand the symptoms seen after abdominal surgery, although the medication and settings of cause will influence the outcome to a large extent.

PAIN FOLLOWING ABDOMINAL SURGERY—WHAT DO WE KNOW?

Changes in the Referred Pain Area

Several studies have explored the pain following acute clinical visceral lesions that share mechanisms with pain after surgery. Giamberardino et al. investigated a series of patients with acute visceral pain (symptomatic renal/ureteral calculosis) and found that pain thresholds to electrical stimulation were found to be significantly lower than normal in the referred pain area corresponding to the deep tissues.[26] Later they investigated patients treated with extracorporeal shock wave lithotripsy where patients demonstrated hyperalgesia in the skin, subcutaneous and muscular tissue in the referred pain area. The hyperalgesia decreased after treatment reflecting a reversal of central sensitization.[25] We took this further to look at patients with acute appendicitis and acute cholecystitis, and found skin hyperalgesia in the somatic referred pain area, but not in the control area.[50,51] The trophic alterations in the deep tissues as demonstrated by the Italian group are more up to discussion. Hence, in a study using both ultrasound and computerized tomography in patients with renal stones, we were not able to reproduce these findings in the deep tissue.[43] In the clinical settings, referred pain to somatic structures is well known after surgery, and the hyperalgesia may explain some of the remote allodynia and pain experienced by these patients; however, controlled studies are still lacking.

Neuronal changes in the referred pain areas have also been investigated after surgery as disorders like the postcholecystectomy syndrome could be a consequence of plastic neuronal changes that in some patients could be irreversible. In some support, Pedersen et al.[43] studied patients with painful stones in the renal pelvis and found that *after the operation* there was a tendency toward increase in the pain thresholds for both single and repeated electrical stimuli in the referred pain area (the affected flank). On the other hand, the pain thresholds on the contralateral (control) site were unaltered after surgery. Brandsborg et al.[12] studied 90 women undergoing hysterectomy for benign conditions and found that cutaneous and vaginal hypersensitivity was associated with acute pain after hysterectomy. The relationship between the sensory changes and persistent pain was less clear, although preoperative brush-evoked allodynia was associated with pelvic pain after 4 months. The study supports previous studies showing that preoperative pain and skin hypersensitivity is related to early postoperative pain the first week after abdominal surgery, whereas the relation to persistent pain is less clear.[1,6,27,30,42,53]

The long-term changes were investigated by Kjaer et al.,[33] who tested 40 patients with quantitative sensory testing (QST) in the referred pain area and in a control area on the contralateral side of the abdomen before and 2 to 7 years after laparoscopic cholecystectomy. Unexpectedly, the initial hypersensitivity in the referred pain area (that was found before surgery[50]) returned to normal in the follow-up period, and also there were no differences in the five patients with postcholecystectomy syndrome. Hence, the neuroplastic changes seen before surgery seem to disappear after successful surgery. The prevalence of postcholecystectomy syndrome was also lower than previously reported, and likely the minimal invasive procedures are responsible for the findings. In conclusion, minor surgery with modern techniques does not seem to provide a permanent change in the referred pain areas. This is in contrast to the robust changes in the referred pain area in chronic abdominal pain disorders. Hence, increased and abnormal referred pain areas were seen in patients with functional chest pain and functional dyspepsia. Furthermore, patients with erosive esophagitis had increased referred pain areas selective to heat stimulation, a finding that likely reflects sensitization of afferents with transient receptor potential cation channel receptors.[19] Similarly, in patients with pain due to chronic pancreatitis, increased areas of referred pain to electrical stimulation of the esophagus, stomach, and duodenum was reported as compared to controls.[17] In these patients, the sensitivity in the referred pain to stimuli at various dermatomes was also related to disease severity,[10,11,14] and segmental hyperalgesia at the pancreatic "viscerotome" predicts the response to treatment.[39] More extensive and long-lasting surgical procedures may therefore lead to permanent changes, but whether or not this will be manifested in the referred pain area needs to be explored in more detail.

Plastic Neuronal Changes Immediately After Surgery

Repeated stimulation of the nociceptive system such as seen during surgery may sensitize the pain system. This may be the initial factor to start a cascade of events as preclinical studies of visceral diseases indicate that they, to a higher degree than somatic tissue lesions, result in central sensitization that does not revert to normal state.[40] Furthermore, there is a tendency for the sensitization to spread to other spinal and supraspinal structures. Therefore, surgery may predispose to a generalized sensitization that lowers the pain threshold in general and serve as a preconditioning factor to pain chronification. Actually, pain after surgery can be seen as an "experimental model" as the painful event is planned and controlled, and therefore the changes in the pain system can be followed systematically. It is well known that certain factors predispose to complications after surgery, and postoperative pain and hyperalgesia is seen more often in patients with preoperative pain and/or stress symptoms.[54,56] On the other hand, in some patients the initial changes in pain processing after the acute trauma *per se* may predict chronic pain. Hence, postoperatively there may be a lowering of the pain threshold after 24 hours, not only at the site of incision but also at remote sites such as the arm or leg (representing generalized sensitivity).[34,55] In those patients who develop chronic pain at 6 months after surgery, more skin and deep tissue hyperalgesia peri-incisionally and distant to the lesion was shown, whereas the clinical pain did not predict pain chronification.[54] In this line, we recently showed that early postoperative hyperalgesia to pressure stimulation 5 days after mamma surgery was an independent risk factor for development of chronic pain after breast cancer surgery.[52] Therefore, the initial response in the nociceptive system with an assessment of whether or not this show pathologic tendencies (lowering of pain thresholds with generalization to remote areas assessed with QST) may predict whether or not pain develops to a chronic state. Longitudinal studies are naturally needed, but on the other hand if proven, the sensitization assessed with QST may serve as a biomarker for chronic postoperative pain.

Persistent Postsurgical Pain and How to Prevent It

Other factors such as the pain response the first week after surgery,[7] the variability in the patients' ability to modulate pain, as well as pain catastrophizing may be clinically relevant for the disposition to acquire pain. Hence, higher levels of preoperative pain catastrophizing have been associated with higher postoperative pain ratings.[28] A general review of the different factors and how they may or may not predict persistent pain is outside the scope of this chapter and the reader is referred to studies of Lavand'hommes[35] and Kehlet et al.[32] However, it is important to stress that the consequences will be to:

1. identify patients at risk (e.g., pre-existing pain, addictive behavior, comorbid stress symptoms, catastrophizing, and depression).

2. assess the evolution of the nociceptive system with QST as outlined in the previous section, as clinical pain complaints may not be useful to predict who will develop chronic pain.
3. consider red flags for sensitization after surgery: (QST shows widespread hyperalgesia, increased temporal summation to repeated stimuli, deficient conditioned pain modulations, and/or less habituation to repeated stimuli) pathologic and intense description of pain and unexplained postprandial pain.
4. treatment: (a) intensify treatment in patients that have evidence for pathologic pain (or where there is high likelihood that they will develop it) using drugs against hyperalgesia such as ketamine and gabapentinoids[10]; (b) use serotonin/norepinephrine reuptake inhibitors (SNRIs)/tapentadol/clonidine when deficient descending control is suspected[37,38,58]; (c) consider epidural/spinal analgesia that reduces the risk for spreading hyperalgesia, if possible[35]; and (d) use opioids carefully and consider that hyperalgesia can easily develop in patients with generalized pain and sensitization.[10]

CONCLUSION

Pain and other symptoms following gastrointestinal surgery can partly be explained from our knowledge of how the visceral pain system responds in other settings. This can be investigated with preclinical, experimental human and clinical studies. However, more persistent changes of the nervous system that may lead to chronic pain syndromes is often more complex and involves psychological factors, comedication, and concomitant pain from other structures. Experimental models, especially, has made it possible to study the plasticity of the pain system the days after surgery, and may contribute to predict which patients are at risk for developing more permanent changes. Such patients are likely candidates for thorough monitoring and intensified treatment to prevent persistent plastic changes of the pain system as a consequence chronic pain.

REFERENCES

1. Aasvang E, Kehlet H. Chronic postoperative pain: the case of inguinal herniorrhaphy. *Br J Anaesth.* 2005;95(1):69–76.
2. Andrews PL, Sanger GJ. Abdominal vagal afferent neurones: an important target for the treatment of gastrointestinal dysfunction. *Curr Opin Pharmacol.* 2002;2(6): 650–656.
3. Arendt-Nielsen L, Laursen RJ, Drewes AM. Referred pain as an indicator for neural plasticity. *Prog Brain Res.* 2000;129:343–356.
4. Arendt-Nielsen L, Yarnitsky D. Experimental and clinical applications of quantitative sensory testing applied to skin, muscles and viscera. *J Pain.* 2009;10(6):556–572.
5. Bielefeldt K, Christianson JA, Davis BM. Basic and clinical aspects of visceral sensation: transmission in the CNS. *Neurogastroenterol Motil.* 2005;17(4):488–499.
6. Bisgaard T, Rosenberg J, Kehlet H. From acute to chronic pain after laparoscopic cholecystectomy: a prospective follow-up analysis. *Scand J Gastroenterol.* 2005;40(11):1358–1364.
7. Blichfeldt-Eckhardt MR, Ørding H, Andersen C, Licht PB, Toft P. Early visceral pain predicts chronic pain after laparoscopic. *Pain.* 2014;155(11):2400–2407.
8. Bouhassira D, Chollet R, Coffin B, et al. Inhibition of a somatic nociceptive reflex by gastric distention in humans. *Gastroenterology.* 1994;107(4):985–992.
9. Bouhassira D, Sabate JM, Coffin B, Le Bars D, Willer JC, Jian R. Effects of rectal distensions on nociceptive flexion reflexes in humans. *Am J Physiol.* 1998;275(3 Pt 1):G410–G417.
10. Bouwense SAW, de Vries M, Schreuder L, et al. Systematic mechanism orientated approach to chronic pancreatitis pain. *World J Gastroenterol.* 2015;21(1):47–59.
11. Bouwense SAW, Olesen SS, Drewes AM, Frøkjær JB, van Goor H, Wilder-Smith OHG. Is altered central pain processing related to disease stage in chronic pancreatitis patients with pain? An exploratory study. *PLoS One.* 2013;8(2):e55460.
12. Brandsborg B, Dueholm M, Kehlet H, Jensen TS, Nikolajsen L. Mechanosensitivity before and after hysterectomy: a prospective study on the prediction of acute and chronic postoperative pain. *Br J Anaesthesia.* 2011;107(6):940–947.
13. Brock C, Andresen T, Frokjaer JB, et al. Central pain mechanisms following combined acid and capsaicin perfusion of the human oesophagus. *Eur J Pain.* 2010;14(3):273–281.
14. Buscher HC, Wilder-Smith OH, van Goor H. Chronic pancreatitis patients show hyperalgesia of central origin: a pilot study. *Eur J Pain.* 2006;10(4):363–370.
15. Cervero F, Connell LA, Lawson SN. Somatic and visceral primary afferents in the lower thoracic dorsal root ganglia of the cat. *J Comp Neurol.* 1984;228(3):422–431.

16. Costa M, Brookes SJ. The enteric nervous system. *Am J Gastroenterol.* 1994;89(8 Suppl): S129–S137.

17. Dimcevski G, Sami SA, Funch-Jensen P, et al. Pain in chronic pancreatitis: the role of reorganization in the central nervous system. *Gastroenterology.* 2007;132(4):1546–1556.

18. Drewes AM, Gregersen H, Arendt-Nielsen L. Experimental pain in gastroenterology: a reappraisal of human studies. *Scand J Gastroenterol.* 2003;38(11):1115–1130.

19. Drewes AM, Reddy H, Pedersen J, Funch-Jensen P, Gregersen H, Arendt-Nielsen L. Multimodal pain stimulations in patients with grade B oesophagitis. *Gut.* 2006;55(7): 926–932.

20. Drewes AM, Schipper KP, Dimcevski G, et al. Multi-modal induction and assessment of allodynia and hyperalgesia in the human oesophagus. *Eur J Pain.* 2003;7:81–91.

21. Drewes AM, Schipper KS, Dimcevski G, et al. Multimodal assessment of pain in the oesophagus: a new experimental model. *Am J Physiol Gastrointest Liver Physiol.* 2002;283(1):G95–G103.

22. Frøkjaer JB, Andersen SD, Gale J, Arendt-Nielsen L, Gregersen G, Drewes AM. An experimental study of viscero-visceral hyperalgesia using an ultrasound-based multimodal sensory testing approach. *Pain.* 2005;119(1–3):191–200.

23. Garrison DW, Chandler MJ, Foreman RD. Viscerosomatic convergence onto feline spinal neurons from esophagus, heart and somatic fields: effects of inflammation. *Pain.* 1992;49(3):373–382.

24. Giamberardino MA, Costantini R, Affaitati G, et al. Viscero-visceral hyperalgesia: characterization in different clinical models. *Pain.* 2010;151(2):307–322.

25. Giamberardino MA, de Bigontina P, Martegiani C, Vecchiet L. Effects of extracorporeal shock-wave lithotripsy on referred hyperalgesia from renal/ureteral calculosis. *Pain.* 1994;56(1):77–83.

26. Giamberardino MA. Recent and forgotten aspects of visceral pain. *Eur J Pain.* 1999; 3(2):77–92.

27. Granot M, Lowenstein L, Yarnitsky D, Tamir A, Zimmer EZ. Postcesarean section pain prediction by preoperative experimental pain assessment. *Anesthesiology.* 2003;98(6): 1422–1426.

28. Grosen K, Drewes AM, Pilegaard HK, Pfeiffer-Jensen M, Brock B, Vase L. Situational but not dispositional pain catastrophizing predict postoperative pain in patients without pain prior to surgery. *J Pain.* 2016;17(5):549–560.

29. Heinricher MM, Tavares I, Leith JL, Lumb BM. Descending control of nociception: specificity, recruitment and plasticity. *Brain Res Rev.* 2009;60(1):214–225.

30. Hsu YW, Somma J, Hung YC, Tsai PS, Yang CH, Chen CC. Predicting postoperative pain by preoperative pressure pain assessment. *Anesthesiology.* 2005;103(3):613–618.

31. Janig W. Neurobiology of visceral afferent neurons: neuroanatomy, functions, organ regulations and sensations. *Biol Psychol.* 1996;42(1–2):29–51.

32. Kehlet H, Jensen TS, Woolf CJ. Persistent postsurgical pain: risk factors and prevention. *Lancet.* 2006;367(9522):1618–1625.

33. Kjaer DW, Stawowy M, Arendt-Nielsen L, Drewes AM, Funch-Jensen P. Reversibility of central neuronal changes in patients recovering from gallbladder stones or acute cholecystitis. *World J Gastroenterol.* 2006;12(46):7522–7526.

34. Lavand'hommes P, De Kock M, Waterloos H. Intraoperative epidural analgesia combined with ketamine provides effective analgesia in patients undergoing major digestive surgery. *Anesthesiology.* 2005;103(4):813–820.

35. Lavand'hommes P. Prevention of pain persistence: anesthesiological aspects. In: Wilder-Smith O, Arendt-Nielsen L, Yarnitsky D, Vissers KCP, eds. *Postoperative Pain.* IASP Press; 2015:201–209.

36. Mayer EA, Aziz Q, Coen S, et al. Brain imaging approaches to the study of functional GI disorders: a Rome working team report. *Neurogastroenterol Motil.* 2009;21(6): 579–596.

37. Neil MJE. Clonidine: clinical pharmacology and therapeutic use in pain management. *Cur Clin Pharmacol.* 2011;6(4):280–287.

38. Niesters M, Proto PL, Aarts L, Sarton EY, Drewes AM, Dahan A. Tapentadol potentiates descending pain inhibition in chronic pain patients with diabetic polyneuropathy. *Br J Anaesth.* 2014;113(1):148–156.

39. Olesen SS, Graversen C, Bouwense SAW, van Goor H, Wilder-Smith OHG, Drewes AM. Quantitative sensory testing predicts pregabalin efficacy in painful chronic pancreatitis. *PLoS One.* 2013;8(3):e57963.

40. Olivar T, Laird JM. Differential effects of N-methyl-D-aspartate receptor blockade on nociceptive somatic and visceral reflexes. *Pain.* 1999;79(1):67–73.

41. Oudenhove LV. Understanding gut-brain interactions in gastrointestinal pain by neuroimaging: lessons from somatic pain studies. *Neurogastroenterol Motil.* 2011;23(4): 292–302.

42. Pan PH, Coghill R, Houle TT, et al. Multifactorial preoperative predictors for postcesarean section pain and analgesic requirement. *Anesthesiology.* 2006;104(3):417–425.

43. Pedersen KV, Drewes AM, Graumann O, et al. Somatosensory and trophic findings in the referred pain area in patients with kidney stone disease. *Scand J Pain.* 2013;4(3):165–170.

44. Qin C, Malykhina AP, Akbarali HI, Foreman RD. Cross-organ sensitization of lumbosacral spinal neurons receiving urinary bladder input in rats with inflamed colon. *Gastroenterology.* 2005;129(6):1967–1978.

45. Ren K, Randich A, Gebhart GF. Effects of electrical stimulation of vagal afferents on spinothalamic tract cells in the rat. *Pain.* 1991;44(3):311–319.

46. Sami SA, Rossel P, Dimcevski G, et al. Cortical changes to experimental sensitization of the human esophagus. *Neuroscience.* 2006;140(1):269–279.

47. Schleim S, Roiser JP. FMRI in translation: the challenges facing real-world applications. *Front Hum Neurosci.* 2009;3:63.

48. Sengupta JN, Gebhart GF. Gastrointestinal afferent fibers and sensation. In: Johnson L, ed. *Physiology of the Gastrointestinal Tract.* New York: Raven Press; 1994:483–519.

49. Sharma A, Lelic D, Brock C, Paine P, Aziz Q. New technologies to investigate the brain-gut axis. *World J Gastroenterol.* 2009;15(2):182–191.

50. Stawowy M, Bluhme C, Arendt-Nielsen L, Drewes AM, Funch-Jensen P. Somatosensory changes in the referred pain area in patients with acute cholecystitis before and after treatment with laparoscopic or open cholecystectomy. *Scand J Gastroenterol.* 2004;39(10):988–993.

51. Stawowy M, Rössel P, Bluhme C, Funch-Jensen P, Arendt-Nielsen L, Drewes AM. Somatosensory changes in the referred pain area following acute inflammation of the appendix. *Eur J Gastroenterol Hepatol.* 2002;14(10):1–6.

52. van Helmond N, Steegers MA, Filippini-de Moor GP, Vissers KC, Wilder-Smith OH. Hyperalgesia and persistent pain after breast cancer surgery: a prospective randomized controlled trial with perioperative COX-2 inhibition. *PLoS One.* 2016;11(12):e0166601.

53. Werner MU, Duun P, Kehlet H. Prediction of postoperative pain by preoperative nociceptive responses to heat stimulation. *Anesthesiology.* 2004;100(1):115–119.

54. Wilder-Smith OHG. Altered perioperative pain processing and persistent pain after surgery. In: Wilder-Smith O, Arendt-Nielsen L, Yarnitsky D, Vissers KCP, eds. *Postoperative Pain.* IASP Press; 2015:149–158.

55. Wilder-Smith OHG, Tassonyi E, Senly C, Otten P, Arendt-Nielsen L. Surgical pain is followed not only by spinal sensitization but also by supraspinal antinociception. *Br J Anaesth.* 1996;76(6):816–821.

56. Wilder-Smith OHG, Chronic pain and surgery: a review of new insights from sensory testing. *J Pain Palliat Care Pharmacother.* 2011;25(2):146–159.

57. Willis WD, Westlund KN. Neuroanatomy of the pain system and of the pathways that modulate pain. *J Clin Neurophysiol.* 1997;14(1):2–31.

58. Yarnitsky D, Granot M, Nahman-Averbuch H, Khamaisi M, Granovsky Y. Conditioned pain modulation predicts duloxetine efficacy in painful diabetic neuropathy. *Pain.* 2012;153(6):1193–1198.

CHAPTER 5

Pain Derived from Gynecologic Laparoscopy

John Jarrell

Pain resulting from pelvic surgery is very common and yet existing reviews of chronic postsurgical pain (CPSP) have not included this type of surgery.[30] One possible explanation may be the fact that many laparoscopic procedures are done to treat pre-existing painful conditions indicated for nonacute pain as well as acute problems. This is a relative contraindication from the criteria proposed by Macrae and Davies.[35] Another factor may be due to the process of health record coding that may miss most of the gynecologic procedures that are ambulatory not associated with hospital admission.[13] One condition related to abdominal visceral surgery that is an exception is cholecystectomy that has a substantial literature on postoperative pain, possibly due to inpatient admissions. Table 5-1 indicates the comparative results of queries in the PubMed and PubMed Central databases published by procedure in relation to CPSP undertaken in May, 2017. Citations of CPSP are dominated by nonpelvic disorders and the majority of pelvic causes are associated with the treatment of endometriosis.

The objective of this chapter is briefly to review the general subject of pain following surgery, gynecologic laparoscopy and pain, visceral pain sensitization, and insight into persistent pain that follows gynecologic laparoscopy.

TABLE 5-1 Publications Regarding ([Postsurgical] and Pain) with Specific Procedures

Procedure	PubMed Central	PubMed
Cholecystectomy	443	36
Hip surgery	1,107	71
Knee surgery	1,259	139
Spine surgery	1,104	157
Breast surgery	1,109	89
Gynecologic laparoscopy	175	13
Endometriosis laparoscopy	102	8
Dated May 14, 2017		

GENERAL REVIEW OF CHRONIC POSTSURGICAL PAIN

The first report considering CPSP was in 1998 and indicated the frequency of the condition was 22.3% in a chronic pain clinic.[12] The most common sites of pain were the abdomen, anus, perineum, and genital areas. Ten years later the same group reported that the possible numbers of cases of CPSP in the United Kingdom were possibly as high as 7,125,000 for the year 2005 to 2006.[34] More recent reviews found similar rates.[9]

The definition of postsurgical pain was first proposed by Macrae: (1) pain develops after a surgical procedure, (2) the duration is at least 2 months, (3) other causes are excluded, (4) pain from a pre-existing condition is excluded.[35] The major procedures associated with postoperative pain included thoracic surgery, hernia, amputation, cardiac surgery, hip replacement, cholecystectomy, and Caesarian section.[11]

The estimated frequency of persistent postsurgical pain is in the range of 10% to 50%.[29] This study emphasized that a measurable portion of these cases can become chronic, that in many cases are due to potentially preventable iatrogenic causes such as nerve injury and undertreated acute severe postoperative pain.[29] In addition, risk factors for the development of CPSP have stressed high rates of preoperative pain and acute pain following surgery.[37] Younger patients are at increased risk of pain following hernia repair, but older individuals are at greater risk of pain from shoulder arthroscopy.[41,43] Women have been identified as being at particular risk for many clinical pain conditions and possibly postsurgical postprocedural pain.[16] Nerve injury is recognized as a prominent risk factor. This specific mechanism of pain development—a nerve injury—is now being considered as a more complicated neuropathic injury that encompasses additional risk factors leading to chronicity.[36] Psychological studies of chronic pain after surgery have focused primarily on anxiety and catastrophizing characteristics in adults. In the pediatric group, factors responsible for the development of chronic pain are different from those contributing to the persistence of pain.[38] Genetic predisposition has been proposed as an important predictor of postoperative pain.[5,47] More recent studies have suggested a mechanism for the development of persistent pain lies in understanding the physiology of pain sensitization.[3,44,51]

A recent review of surgically induced neuropathic pain has provided a phased approach to the establishment of persistent postoperative pain that includes a comprehensive view of patient-related factors, the surgical incision, approaches to the measurement of pain experience, and measures to prevent its development.[7] While this is a comprehensive approach to postoperative pain, it does not actually reference the specific type of tissue that is involved in the surgery as a variable. In the present chapter, these concepts will be expanded to include a consideration of the tissues involved in the surgical procedure—specifically, pelvic visceral tissues.

GYNECOLOGIC LAPAROSCOPY

One of the most common procedures undertaken in the field of gynecology is operative laparoscopy in the diagnosis and management of acute and chronic pelvic pain. Ambulatory gynecologic procedures rank fifth in ambulatory procedures following gastrointestinal; ocular; ear, nose, and throat; musculoskeletal; and neurosurgical procedures.[13] In the period 1994 to 1996, there were more than 350,000 ambulatory laparoscopic procedures in the United States.[48]

Laparoscopy is undertaken for both acute and nonacute conditions. In the former situation, the diagnosis is usually apparent: hemorrhage emanating from an ectopic pregnancy or ruptured ovarian cyst, inflammation from pelvic infection or mechanical torsion of a visceral structure. In nonacute situations, however, there is less specificity in many cases regarding the pathology involved that is causing pain and as a consequence the results of surgery are less successful than in the acute emergency.[6,20] The procedure is commonly undertaken for nonacute conditions such the diagnosis and treatment of potentially neoplastic cysts, adhesions, and endometriosis lesions. It is further complicated as there are often multiple procedures undertaken in the same operation. The common feature of these procedures is that they involve tissue injury to somatic and visceral tissues.

LIMITATIONS OF LAPAROSCOPIC SURGERY FOR PAIN

The Negative Laparoscopy

There are several important limitations in the treatment of nonacute problems. In many instances, there are no identifiable lesions in the pelvis and the procedure is termed "negative." The reported incidence of a negative laparoscopy varies greatly as shown in Table 5-2.[10,14,31] The impact on the woman may be one of reassurance but also dismay that there is no identifiable lesion causing her pain. There can be significant disappointment that there is no definitive diagnosis due to high levels of expectation that the symptoms are characteristic of endometriosis. As a result, this can be particularly upsetting if the woman is simply told that "nothing was found" similar to the problems faced in functional

TABLE 5-2 **Reported Rates "Negative" Laparoscopy**

Author	Year	Reported Sample	% Negative Laparoscopy	Source
Drozgyik	2007	1,061	29.5	*J Obstet Gynecol Reprod Biol*
Johnson	2004	123	45.5	*BJOG*. 111(9):950
Levitan	1985	186	92	*Int J Obstet Gynecol*
Howard	1996	521	35	*JAAGL*. 4(1):85–94
Carter	1994	141	0	*JAAGL*. 2(1):43–47

pain conditions like fibromyalgia and whiplash. Although some have indicated that the rate of "negative laparoscopy" should, with appropriate clinical examination, be a rare finding, others have indicated this is a common experience. It has been suggested there may be invisible endometriosis associated with severe pain although there are no data to support the removal of microscopic endometriosis with improvement in pain. One of the most common conditions associated with a negative laparoscopy is that of dysmenorrhea. This condition is commonly overlooked as it can erroneously be considered a side effect of a normal physiologic process. Dysmenorrhea is very common among women with chronic pelvic pain—approaching 70% overall and 90% among women with verified pain sensitization. The condition is self-reported and only recently have there been attempts to categorize women with dysmenorrhea by severity. Cohorts of women with endometriosis have been shown to be virtually identical to women who experienced a negative laparoscopy, both in terms of not only pain severity, duration, and demographics, but also in tests of pain sensitization as is discussed below. A recent comparison of women with negative laparoscopy versus women with confirmed endometriosis has shown the groups to be essentially identical in demographic, clinical, and pain testing results.[24] This would suggest the cause of the pain and pain sensitization may be, for example, the uterus. This is consistent with reports of neural tissues within the endometrium of women with and without endometriosis.[1]

Limited Benefit of Surgery

There is also increasing awareness of the limited benefit of treating laparoscopically early endometriosis.[27] In addition, virtually all gynecologists have experienced the observation that endometriosis was successfully cauterized or excised with apparent improvement in the woman's symptoms for about 6 months when the pain recurs and there is an understandable concern on the part of the woman the "the endometriosis is back." This leads to more frequent and repeated operative laparoscopies.[20] Repeated or revision surgeries and particularly those based solely on the indication pain are known very often to worsen the condition and involved pain.[40,44] One theory that has provided an explanation for the recurrent laparoscopy phenomenon is based now on the recognition of pain relief from inhibition of the neuromuscular junction with botulinum toxin. It is now being considered that the recurrent pain and myofascial hyperalgesia is terminated through the uses of paralytic agents as part of the anesthetic process for operative laparoscopy. It may take a number of months for the recurrent hyperalgesia to recur. Many women present with severe pain 6 months following surgery due to the recurrence of hyperalgesia from abdominal wall trigger points.

Although there is a myriad of citations associated with the procedure to remove various aspects of endometriosis, there are very few studies associated with the frequency of repeated laparoscopy.[15,21,49] One such study measuring the entire provincial experience in the Province of Alberta during the period 1994/95 to 2005/06 did identify the frequency of operative and diagnostic laparoscopy among a total of 24,896 procedures. The repeat rates of operative laparoscopy by individual woman were 36%: two or more operative procedures, 13%: three or more, 5%: four or more, and 2%: five or more procedures.[21] The use of measures of repeat procedures within a 1-year period fluctuated significantly, demonstrating significant variation.[20]

Is there an explanation for these challenges to laparoscopic surgery for pain? On the one hand, there is significant pain in the absence of pathology and on the other hand there is limited benefit from the removal of existing pathology. Is there a common denominator explanation for these two apparently conflicting observations?

Pain Sensitization—Detectable Preoperatively but Invisible at Laparoscopy

Increasingly pain sensitization is being recognized as a condition that can contribute to an erroneous attribution to and misinterpretation of the cause of pain at the time of surgery. Sensitization is deemed peripheral when there is increased responsiveness and reduced threshold of stimulated nociceptive neurons in the periphery. Central sensitization is increased responsiveness of nociceptive neurons in the central nervous system to their normal or subthreshold afferent input. This may be attributed to increased pain responses in pain patients where an ongoing neuronal barrage of the central neurons may trigger a sensitization process. Sensitization may be due to visible conditions in the pelvis such as endometriosis but can also be caused by severe dysmenorrhea (repeated painful attacks), in which the surgical assessment may indicate no obvious and known pathology. The presence of sensitization is only indirectly appreciated by clinical quantitative pain testing indicating hyperalgesia or allodynia.

Pain sensitization has been associated with a large number of conditions such as osteoarthritis, fibromyalgia, rheumatoid arthritis, headache, neuropathic pain, temporomandibular pain, complex regional pain, musculoskeletal pain, postsurgical pain, and a variety of visceral pain syndromes.[50] It has been shown that repeated surgeries further enhance the sensitization. The relationship of endometriosis to pain sensitization has been reported.[4,45,46]

Visceral pain syndromes resulting in pain sensitization also include dysmenorrhea.[19] In a review of 185 women with chronic pelvic pain for more than 6 months, the overall prevalence of severe dysmenorrhea was 74%. Among women with sensitization as defined by the presence of allodynia, severe dysmenorrhea was significantly more frequent compared to women without sensitization (89% vs. 68%).[22] Notably sensitization appears to develop over the duration of severe dysmenorrhea. The evaluation of pain sensitization using pressure pain thresholds on the lower abdomen correlated negatively with the years of severe dysmenorrhea.[22]

One condition that closely mimics the issues related to visceral pelvic pain is that of the postcholecystectomy syndrome where there is pain that is similar to when the diseased gall bladder was present.[39] The original observation of allodynia and hyperalgesia in the right upper quadrant of the abdomen was made by Mackenzie in 1913.[33] In addition to the emergence of allodynia as a consequence of biliary colic, he also noted a tender area within the allodynia corresponding to an anterior cutaneous nerve.[33]

The detection of allodynia is based on awareness of the innervation of the pelvic organs by the spinal segments of T10–T12 and L1–L2 as well as the S234 segments. Abdominal allodynia can be identified by drawing a cotton-tipped applicator down the mid-clavicular line along an imaginary line of the lateral border of the rectus muscle bilaterally toward the region where the T12 and L1 nerves would emerge from the anterior rectus sheath.[25] In some instances, the allodynia must first be provoked by placing pressure on these areas. Also, the sensation in some instances is not initially painful but appears to be a paresthesia. Repetitive testing will enhance the pain experience and commonly results in an expansion of the areas of allodynia, presumably from increasing neural activity in the corresponding segments of the spinal cord.[23]

Within the area of allodynia in the region of the T12 and L1 nerves, pain pressure thresholds can be measured using an algometer. The reduction in pressure pain threshold is an indicator of pain sensitization. The identification of reduced pressure pain thresholds permits further objective confirmation of the central sensitization.[22] It is interesting that sensitized women commonly complain of an inability to wear tight jeans and lie on their stomachs presumably due to the lower abdominal hyperalgesia and allodynia. An example of this common finding, the location of allodynia and the tender points on the abdomen is presented in Figure 5-1.

Unfortunately, with the recurrence of pain after laparoscopic surgery there is a natural inclination to identify the pain with recurrent disease. The hyperalgesia of the lower abdomen from viscero-somatic referral can produce symptoms that are similar to disease involved in the uterus and adnexal disease as was first noted in 1913 by Mackenzie.[32] An alternative explanation to recurrence of endometriosis is that the prior pain experience has been severe enough to alter the nervous system and resulted in a chronic pain sensitization that is not immediately resolved by surgery. This may be one explanation why repeated procedures are not particularly helpful in many cases. The innervation of the pelvic organs is through the sympathetic chain of T10–L1 and the parasympathetic nerves of S2–3–4. Visceral pain is transmitted to these spinal segments through a physiologic mechanism for the brain to identify disturbances in the uterus tubes, ovaries and vagina. The pain from pelvic organs is experienced as diffuse and referred. Under severe pain experience or repeated painful insults such as the presence of severe monthly menstruation or endometriosis deposits, the pain

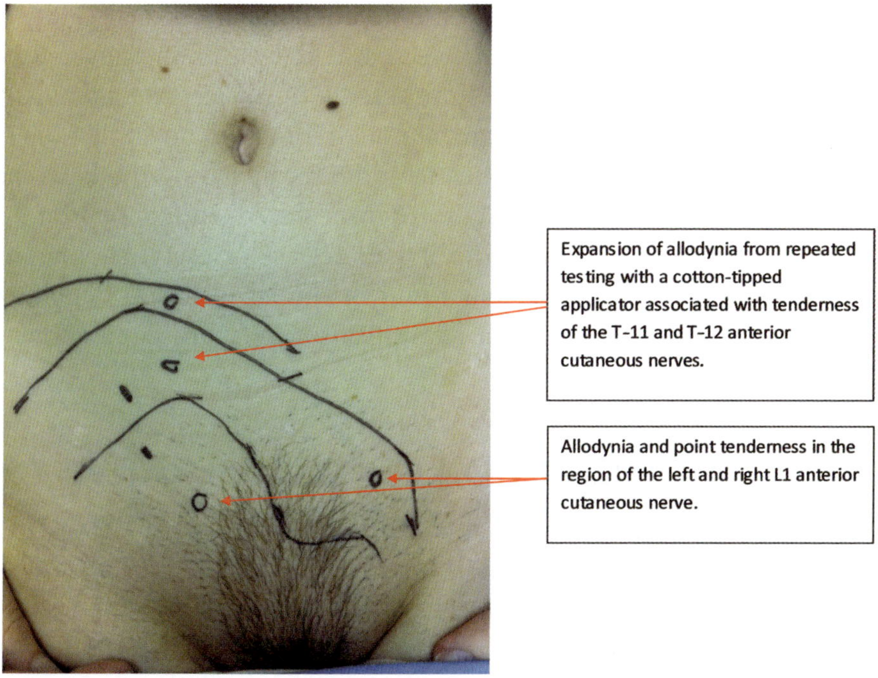

FIGURE 5-1 The pattern of allodynia associated with a woman with chronic pelvic pain associated with primarily a longstanding lesion of the right adnexa. The pattern of allodynia surrounds the anterior cutaneous nerve L1. Similar tenderness in noted in the region of the L1 nerve on the

undergoes viscero-somatic pain referral.[2] This leads to a transmission of the painful stimuli to the pelvic muscles and skin that results in referred somatic allodynia and hyperalgesia.[25] These changes that indicate the presence of sensitization can be detected clinically through simple bedside tests using a tip on the skin of the abdomen and a pressure algometry. The processes of pain are transmitted at least in part by the anterior cutaneous nerves of the abdomen and the pudendal nerves on the perineum.

It is possible that the reason some women improve after laparoscopic surgery is the paralytic agents that are used to intubate the respiratory tract safely. Recent work on the mechanism of action of botulinum toxin on individuals with migraine has suggested there is an inhibitory effect of the neuromuscular junctions of the muscles that are the victim of severe sensitization.[17] The sites used for the injections of botulinum toxin in the management of chronic migraine are similar to the trigger points associated with referred pain. The use of botulinum toxin is now understood to suppress the activity of nociceptive afferents that maintains sensitization of pain although it is also known that the drug has antinociceptive properties in addition, including the blocking of CGRP, glutamate, and substance P from the trigeminal neuron.[18] The actions of botulinum toxin to impair release of acetyl choline at the neuromuscular junction may result in similar effects of depolarizing and nondepolarizing muscle relaxants used in laparoscopic surgery.

THE PREDICTION OF POSTOPERATIVE GYNECOLOGIC LAPAROSCOPY

Preoperative pain testing has been shown to predict postoperative pain in laparoscopic surgery for pelvic visceral disease. Preoperative testing of women having tubal ligations predicted postoperative pain with movement when assessed 10 days postoperatively.[42] Women having a hysterectomy had positive tests for allodynia and pressure pain preoperatively that predicted acute pain after surgery but not 4 months postoperatively.[8]

A study of 71 women having operative laparoscopy for either tubal ligation or nonacute pain were tested pre- and postoperatively for pain, psychosocial tests, and pain testing including cutaneous allodynia, pressure pain thresholds, and trigger points. The psychosocial tests included The Pain Catastrophizing Scale, The Pain Disability Index, the Center for Epidemiology Depression Scale, and the Short Form McGill Pain Questionnaire. As this chapter demonstrates evidence to support the benefits of pain testing, the results will be detailed.[26]

Preoperative average pain was highly correlated with measures of psychosocial health. Surgery resulted in a significant decrease in the average pain and the psychosocial tests.[28] There was a greater effect of the change in average pain and psychosocial testing in the presence of preoperative allodynia. Women with positive pain tests for sensitization also had higher average pain at baseline than those with negative findings and were seen to have a greater reduction in average pain when assessed at six months after surgery.[28] A regression analysis demonstrated that postoperative pain could be predicted preoperatively from the presence of allodynia, catastrophizing and the baseline avert gauge pan. The presence of sensitization was shown to be an independent factor in the prediction of postoperative pain.[26,28]

RELATIONSHIP OF PREOPERATIVE PAIN TESTING TO THE SURGICAL PROCEDURES

The frequency of positive pain testing was similar pre- and postoperatively among those having surgery for nonacute pain. However, there was a change in the distribution as some individuals lost sensitization, some gained sensitization and others did not note a difference (Fig. 5-1). Twenty-six women tested positive preoperatively; 9 became pain free and 17 had persistent pain at 6 months. Ten of these women had an elimination of positive tests for sensitization. The women who lost the sensitization had the greatest reduction in average pain (Fig. 5-2).

Twenty women who tested negatively for sensitization preoperatively had a lower reduction in average pain postoperatively than that

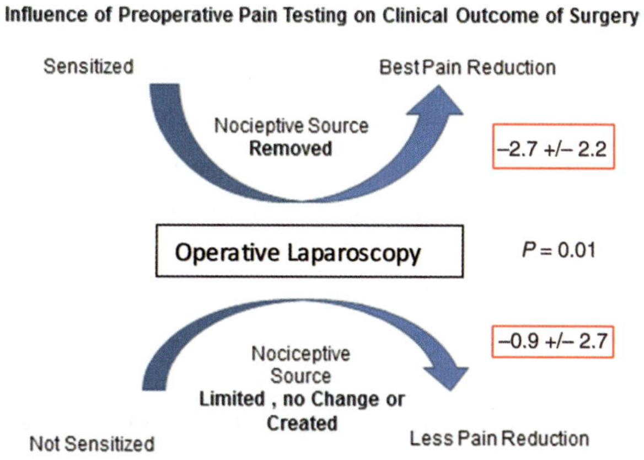

FIGURE 5-2 Visual depiction of changes in pain postoperatively among women with changes in preoperative sensitization testing. Success is associated with identification and removal of the nociceptive source.

seen when there was sensitization. Further, while 17 remained negative, sensitization developed at 6 months in 7. The women who developed sensitization after surgery had a lowest pain reduction postoperatively (Fig. 5-2).

This study indicated that changes in the presence of sensitization from pre- to postoperative assessment may be a further variable in the assessment of success of surgery. The loss or gain in pain sensitivity testing was associated with changes in average pain supporting the role of preoperative testing. This association appears to suggest that the results of surgery on pelvic visceral tissues are dependent on the presence and degree of nociceptive activity emerging from lesions in the operative field. Viscerally related surgery may result in changes in pain that differ somewhat from the neutrally mediated pain associated with more somatic-related tissue.

WHAT ARE THE PRACTICAL IMPLICATIONS OF PAIN SENSITIZATION IN GYNECOLOGIC SURGERY?

- Preoperative sensory testing provides an opportunity to recognize the possibility of a negative laparoscopy, inform the patient of such, and broaden the discussion to alternative causes such as dysmenorrhea. Preoperative testing can inform the patient of the possibility that there may be an improvement in pain if the structure that is being removed is the source of nociception.
- Preoperative and postoperative testing provides an objective test to support improvement in the clinical condition.

Quantitative sensitization testing can provide a way to demonstrate objectively what is a complaint based entirely on self-report. The testing is a validating exercise for a woman who may in many cases have received only negative responses to the complaints as there is no evidence of anything more serious than a side effect from a physiologic process.

There are practical benefits to the identification of pain sensitization both when there is a visible lesion and when none is identified. With a visible lesion, the presence of sensitization is a clinical marker for objective improvement from the removal of the nociceptive focus. Preoperative sensitization has been shown to predict improvement postoperatively, presumably from the removal of the initiating pathology. When no visible lesion is identified at laparoscopy the identification of sensitization validates the woman's complaint and reduces stress associated with the comment that nothing was found. It may also lead to the recognition of alternative causes for sensitization, most commonly severe dysmenorrhea but may also include irritable bowel disease and interstitial cystitis.

CONCLUSION

The exact incidence of chronic pain following laparoscopy has not been determined. On one study of 270 women with chronic pelvic pain, the incidence of prior laparoscopy was 46%. In summary, the causes of postoperative pain following gynecologic laparoscopy appear to be related to either the presence of undetermined dysmenorrhea or the persistence or emergence of severe pain sensitization from prior pain states or alternatively may be developed from the surgical insult itself. The benefit of quantitative sensory tests permits an ability to categorize chronic pain patients based on severity, appreciate the morbidity of the condition, and have objective means to follow the effectiveness of treatment. Furthermore, it will provide information on how vulnerable the patient is for surgery. The value of these clinical tests, the ease of bedside testing, and the ability to provide an alternative explanation for the pelvic pain can contribute to the diagnostic accuracy of women having surgery for nonacute pelvic pain.

REFERENCES

1. Al-Jefout M, Dezarnaulds G, Cooper M, et al. Diagnosis of endometriosis by detection of nerve fibres in an endometrial biopsy: a double blind study. *Hum Reprod*. 2009; 24(12):3019–3024.
2. Arendt-Nielsen L, Schipper KP, Dimcevski G, et al. Viscero-somatic reflexes in referred pain areas evoked by capsaicin stimulation of the human gut. *Eur J Pain*. 2008;12(5):544–551.

3. Baert IA, Lluch E, Mulder T, Nijs J, Noten S, Meeus M. Does pre-surgical central modulation of pain influence outcome after total knee replacement? A systematic review. *Osteoarthritis Cartilage*. 2016;24(2):213–223.
4. Bajaj P, Bajaj P, Madsen H, Arendt-Nielsen L. Endometriosis is associated with central sensitization: a psychophysical controlled study. *J Pain*. 2003;4(7):372–380.
5. Belfer I, Dai F, Kehlet H, et al. Association of functional variations in COMT and GCH1 genes with postherniotomy pain and related impairment. *Pain*. 2015;156(2):273–279.
6. Berlanda N, Vercellini P, Fedele L. The outcomes of repeat surgery for recurrent symptomatic endometriosis. *Curr Opin Obstet Gynecol*. 2010;22(4):320–325.
7. Borsook D, Kussman BD, George E, Becerra LR, Burke DW. Surgically induced neuropathic pain: understanding the perioperative process. *Ann Surg*. 2013;257(3):403–412.
8. Brandsborg B, Dueholm M, Kehlet H, Jensen TS, Nikolajsen L. Mechanosensitivity before and after hysterectomy: a prospective study on the prediction of acute and chronic postoperative pain. *Br J Anaesth*. 2011;107(6):940–947.
9. Bruce J, Quinlan J. Chronic post surgical pain. *Rev Pain*. 2011;5(3):23–29.
10. Carter JE. Laparoscopic treatment for chronic pelvic pain: results from three-year follow-up. *J Am Assoc Gynecol Laparosc*. 1994;1(4, Part 2):S6–S7.
11. Costantini R, Affaitati G, Massimini F, Tana C, Innocenti P, Giamberardino MA. Laparoscopic cholecystectomy for gallbladder calculosis in fibromyalgia patients: impact on musculoskeletal pain, somatic hyperalgesia and central sensitization. *PLoS One*. 2016;11(4):e0153408.
12. Crombie IK, Davies HT, Macrae WA. Cut and thrust: antecedent surgery and trauma among patients attending a chronic pain clinic. *Pain*. 1998;76(1–2):167–171.
13. Cullen KA, Hall MJ, Golosinskiy A. Ambulatory surgery in the United States, 2006. US Department of Health and Human Services; 2009. Report No.: 11.
14. Drozgyik I, Vizer M, Szabo I. Significance of laparoscopy in the management of chronic pelvic pain. *Eur J Obstet Gynecol Reprod Biol*. 2007;133(2):223–226.
15. Fedele L, Bianchi S, Zanconato G, Berlanda N, Raffaelli R, Fontana E. Laparoscopic excision of recurrent endometriomas: long-term outcome and comparison with primary surgery. *Fertil Steril*. 2006;85(3):694–699.
16. Fillingim RB, King CD, Ribeiro-Dasilva MC, Rahim-Williams B, Riley JL, 3rd. Sex, gender, and pain: a review of recent clinical and experimental findings. *J Pain*. 2009; 10(5):447–485.
17. Gazerani P, Au S, Dong X, Kumar U, Arendt-Nielsen L, Cairns BE. Botulinum neurotoxin type A (BoNTA) decreases the mechanical sensitivity of nociceptors and inhibits neurogenic vasodilation in a craniofacial muscle targeted for migraine prophylaxis. *Pain*. 2010;151(3):606–616.

18. Gazerani P, Pedersen NS, Staahl C, Drewes AM, Arendt-Nielsen L. Subcutaneous Botulinum toxin type A reduces capsaicin-induced trigeminal pain and vasomotor reactions in human skin. *Pain.* 2009;141(1–2):60–69.
19. Giamberardino MA, Costantini R, Affaitati G, et al. Viscero-visceral hyperalgesia: characterization in different clinical models. *Pain.* 2010;151(2):307–322.
20. Jarrell J. Annual repeat rates of laparoscopic surgery: a marker of practice variation. *Am J Med Qual.* 2010;25(5):378–383.
21. Jarrell J. Diagnostic and operative laparoscopy in Alberta 1994–2006. *J Obstet Gynaecol Can.* 2008;30:1045–1049.
22. Jarrell J, Arendt-Nielsen L. Allodynia and dysmenorrhea. *J Obstet Gynaecol Can.* 2016; 38(3):270–274.
23. Jarrell J, Arendt-Nielsen L. Quantitative sensory testing in gynaecology: improving preoperative and postoperative pain diagnosis. *J Obstet Gynaecol Can.* 2013;35(6):531–535.
24. Jarrell J, Arendt-Nielsen L. The negative laparoscopy unveiled. *J Endometr Pelvic Pain Disord.* 2017; Accepted with minor modifications.
25. Jarrell J, Giamberardino MA, Robert M, Nasr-Esfahani M. Bedside testing for chronic pelvic pain: discriminating visceral from somatic pain. *Pain Res Treat.* 2011;2011:692102.
26. Jarrell J, Giamberardino MA, Robert M, Tang S, Stephanson K. Psychosocial tests, pain sensitization and laparoscopic pelvic surgery. *Scand J Pain.* 2018;18(1):49–57. Accepted November, 2017.
27. Jarrell J, Mohindra R, Ross S, Taenzer P, Brant R. Laparoscopy and reported pain among patients with endometriosis. *J Obstet Gynaecol Can.* 2005;27(5):477–485.
28. Jarrell J, Ross S, Robert M, et al. Prediction of postoperative pain after gynecologic laparoscopy for nonacute pelvic pain. *Am J Obstet Gynecol.* 2014;211(4):360.e1–e8.
29. Kehlet H, Jensen TS, Woolf CJ. Persistent postsurgical pain: risk factors and prevention. *Lancet.* 2006;367(9522):1618–1625.
30. Kissin I, Gelman S. Chronic postsurgical pain: still a neglected topic? *J Pain Res.* 2012;5:473–489.
31. Kresch AJ, Seifer DB, Sachs LB, Barrese I. Laparoscopy in 100 women with chronic pelvic pain. *Obstet Gynecol.* 1984;64(5):672–674.
32. Mackenzie J. Remarks on the meaning and mechanism of visceral pain as shown by the study of visceral and other sympathetic (Autonomic) reflexes. *Br Med J.* 1906; 1(2374):1523–1528.
33. Mackenzie J. *Symptoms and Their Interpretation.* 2nd ed. New York: Paul B Hoeber; 1913.

34. Macrae WA. Chronic post-surgical pain: 10 years on. *Br J Anaesth*. 2008;101(1):77–86.
35. Macrae WA, Davies HT. Chronic postsurgical pain. In: Crombie IK, Linton SJ, Croft PR, Von Korff M, LeReasche L, eds. *Epidemiology of Pain*. Seattle: IASP; 1999: 125–142.
36. Maguire MF, Latter JA, Mahajan R, Beggs FD, Duffy JP. A study exploring the rolelof intercostal nerve damage in chronic pain after thoracic surgery. *Eur J Cardiothorac Surg*. 2006;29(6):873–879.
37. Nikolajsen L, Ilkjaer S, Krøner K, Christensen JH, Jensen TS. The influence of preamputation pain on postamputation stump and phantom pain. *Pain*. 1997;72(3):393–405.
38. Page MG, Watt-Watson J, Choiniere M. Do depression and anxiety profiles over time predict persistent post-surgical pain? A study in cardiac surgery patients. *Eur J Pain*. 2017;21(6):965–976.
39. Persson AK, Dyrehag LE, Akeson J. Prediction of postoperative pain from electrical pain thresholds after laparoscopic cholecystectomy. *Clin J Pain*. 2017;33(2):126–131.
40. Petersen KK, Arendt-Nielsen L, Simonsen O, Wilder-Smith O, Laursen MB. Presurgical assessment of temporal summation of pain predicts the development of chronic postoperative pain 12 months after total knee replacement. *Pain*. 2015;156(1):55–61.
41. Poobalan AS, Bruce J, King PM, Chambers WA, Kruckowski ZH, Smith WC. Chronic pain and quality of life following open inguinal hernia repair. *Br J Surg*. 2001;88(8):1122–1126.
42. Rudin A, Wolner-Hanssen P, Hellbom M, Werner MU. Prediction of post-operative pain after a laparoscopic tubal ligation procedure. *Acta Anaesthesiol Scand*. 2008; 52(7):938–945.
43. SImon CB, Riley JL, 3rd, Coronado RA, et al. Older age as a prognostic factor of attenuated pain recovery after shoulder arthroscopy. *PM R*. 2016;8(4):297–304.
44. Skou ST, Graven-Nielsen T, Rasmussen S, Simonsen OH, Laursen MB, Arendt-Nielsen L. Facilitation of pain sensitization in knee osteoarthritis and persistent post-operative pain: a cross-sectional study. *Eur J Pain*. 2014;18(7):1024–1031.
45. Stratton P, Berkley KJ. Chronic pelvic pain and endometriosis: translational evidence of the relationship and implications. *Hum Reprod Update*. 2011;17(3):327–346.
46. Taylor RN, Hummelshoj L, Stratton P, Vercellini P. Pain and endometriosis: etiology, impact, and therapeutics. *Middle East Fertil Soc J*. 2012;17(4):221–225.
47. Thomazeau J, Rouquette A, Martinez V, et al. Predictive factors of chronic post-surgical pain at 6 months following knee replacement: influence of postoperative pain trajectory and genetics. *Pain Physician*. 2016;19(5):E729–E741.
48. Tu FF, Beaumont JL. Outpatient laparoscopy for abdominal and pelvic pain in the United States 1994 through 1996. *Am J Obstet Gynecol*. 2006;194(3):699–703.

49. Vercellini P, Crosignani PG, Abbiati A, Somigliana E, Vigano P, Fedele L. The effect of surgery for symptomatic endometriosis: the other side of the story. *Hum Reprod Update*. 2009;15(2):177–188.

50. Woolf CJ. Central sensitization: implications for the diagnosis and treatment of pain. *Pain*. 2011;152(3 Suppl):S2–S15.

51. Woolf CJ, Chong MS. Preemptive analgesia–treating postoperative pain by preventing the establishment of central sensitization. *Anesth Analg*. 1993;77(2):362–379.

CHAPTER 6

Vaginal Mesh or Vaginal Mess: Pain and Pelvic Organ Prolapse Surgery

Magali Robert

Pelvic organ prolapse (POP) is the descent of organs through the vagina. It is very common; with up to 50% of women developing prolapse in their lifetime.[17,18] The lifetime risk of a woman undergoing POP surgery is 19%.[31] The prolapse can involve different sites including: descent of the uterus or vault (apical prolapse), the anterior vaginal wall (cystocele), the posterior wall (rectocele and/or enterocele), or any combination thereof. The prolapse may be mild or lead to complete eversion of the vagina exteriorly (procidentia). Once symptomatic, women present with pelvic discomfort worse with activity, feeling of a bulge, and bowel and/or bladder dysfunction. This leads to a significant impact on their quality of life and self-esteem.[20] As the population continues to age, we can expect to see an increase in this already common problem.

Prolapse can be treated conservatively with pelvic floor retraining, in cases of mild prolapse. The use of pessaries (vaginal prostheses) is an option but this requires ongoing surveillance. Surgery is often resorted to after failed conservative management or women's preferences. The aim of surgery is to repair anatomic defects and reposition the vagina to its normal position, thus re-establishing function. Traditionally native tissue repairs have been performed with conflicting successes. The use of synthetic meshes was thought to revolutionize POP surgery. This was spurred by the success of using permanent polypropylene mesh for inguinal hernia repairs. Using mesh for these surgeries has been accepted as the surgery of choice.[11] In addition to increased success rates, overall there was a decrease in persistent pain with the use of mesh over native tissue repair.[11] The use of permanent polypropylene mesh bands for treating urinary stress incontinence was introduced in the late 1990s. The ease of performing the surgery paired with its high success rate resulted in adoption of the procedure as the preferred surgery for urinary stress incontinence. In searching for surgical interventions that could improve success rates, it made inherent sense to use mesh for POP surgery. Since 2005, there was an exponential flurry of new vaginal meshes and mesh kits that flooded the surgical repertoire. This flourished until an FDA warning was issued in October 2008.[13] It stated that adverse events had been reported and may be higher than previously expected and that caution should be used. These complications included mesh extrusions/erosions and pain. In 2011, the FDA issued a follow-up statement that adverse events were not rare as previously thought.[14] This resulted in one of the largest class action medical lawsuits in the United States. The major theme was that women developed chronic pain which then led to a debilitating life.

There are essentially three compartments that can be operated on for prolapse repair: apical, anterior, and posterior. The mesh kits were designed to address the apical and either anterior or posterior compartments. Some mesh kits addressed all compartments. The mesh would fit like a glove around the vagina. The mesh has arms which pass through ligaments to support it. Some kits had anchors to attach to the ligaments. Apically, the attachment was on the sacrospinous ligament medial to the ischial spine. In the anterior compartment, the arms track through the obturator fossa, some kits placing two arms. Posteriorly, the mesh is most often attached apically through the sacrospinous ligament and laid flat in the posterior vagina, although some kits had the mesh traverse the ischiorectal space. Ingrowth of tissue and scarring would hold the mesh (and prolapse) in place.

There are many reasons a woman may have pain following pelvic reconstruction surgery with permanent mesh. She may have had underlying pain, she may have pain following surgery that is not mesh related, and/or she may have a mesh-related complication. Understanding these interplays will elucidate some of the raised concerns and provide guidance for the future. In addition, the management outcomes of pain following surgery should be explored. If the complications are rare but has significant morbidity with poor management outcomes, this would further bring mesh use in question.

BASELINE PAIN

Chronic pelvic pain affects approximately 15% of women in the general population.[38] Its etiology is multifactorial and can include pelvic floor muscle pain (PFMP), interstitial cystitis, endometriosis, pelvic adhesive disease, pelvic congestion syndrome, irritable bowel syndrome, vestibulodynia, pudendal neuralgia, and so forth. Rarely is chronic pelvic pain associated with only POP. However, a woman who has pelvic floor tightness often resorts to straining for evacuation of bladder and bowel. This will predispose her to developing prolapse. In addition, constipation is often a side effect of medications used for the treatment of pain effect which leads to straining and resultant prolapse. Thus the baseline pain levels in women undergoing prolapse surgery are important as it will have a bearing on surgical outcomes. Preoperative pain is a risk factor for postoperative pain (OR: 3.2; 95% CI 1.2–8.4).[37] This is seen in hysterectomy for benign conditions (OR: 2.98; 95% confidence interval [CI], 1.54–5.77)[4] and for inguinal hernia surgery (OR: 2.1; 95% CI, 1.8–2.6).[15]

There are few studies reporting rates of pelvic pain prior to POP surgery. Using the question: "do you experience lower abdominal or genital pain" as a measure of pelvic pain, 25% of preoperative women reported to be at least moderately bothered.[37] Most studies reporting preoperative pain focus on dyspareunia (pain with intercourse). This may be an unreliable marker of pain as the prolapse in and of itself can cause dyspareunia. The rate of dyspareunia preoperatively ranges from 15%

to 25% among sexually active women.[10,35] The cause of the dyspareunia is not further explored recognizing that many potential etiologies will not be improved following prolapse surgery (e.g., atrophy, vulvodynia, painful bladder syndrome/interstitial cystitis, and endometriosis).

The baseline pain prior to surgery is important in evaluating the role of surgery. The paucity of preoperative information makes the results of prospective outcome studies difficult to interpret. Of the few studies that have evaluated baseline pain, it appears that preoperative rates are similar to reports of the general population.

MESH AND PAIN

In a Cochrane review, the authors concluded that any type of mesh augmentation had less recurrent rates of prolapse than native tissue repair (RR 0.53, 95% CI 0.31–0.88, 12 RCTs, $n = 1675$).[25] However, this was at a higher rate of repeat surgery for other complications (RR 2.40, 95% CI 1.51–3.81, 7 RCTs, $n = 867$). These complications included a combination of mesh extrusions and dyspareunia. However, there was no evidence of a difference between the groups in rates of de novo dyspareunia (RR 0.92, 95% CI 0.58–1.47, 11 RCTs, $n = 764$). The rate was 30/389 (7.7%) for mesh compared to 31/375 (8.2%) for native tissue repair. This would seem to indicate that the mesh in and of itself would not be a contributing factor; the surgery, dissection, and healing/scarring would be. The authors do maintain that these results are based on low-quality evidence. Interestingly prospective studies reporting pre- and postoperative dyspareunia (including de novo) often report overall improved rates following surgery.[10,22,27]

In a follow-up, Cochrane review focusing on anterior prolapse repair only, Maher et al.[24] reported no difference in de novo dyspareunia rates with mesh repairs compared to native tissue repairs between 1- and 3-year follow-up. The pooled native tissue repair group had a de novo dyspareunia rate of 11/290 (3.8%) compared to 21/293 (7.2%) for permanent mesh repair (RR 0.54, 95% CI 0.27–1.06). However, once again the quality of evidence was rated as low. There was no difference 1 to 2 years following surgery in the overall dyspareunia rate (which would also include prior pain) (RR 1.06, 95% CI 0.59–1.90). The rates were 19/547 (3.5%) with native repair compared to 18/549 (3.3%) with the mesh group. Overall pain (pelvic) was reported in only one study.[9] It was reported as 18% in the mesh group compared with 9% in the native tissue repair group (nonsignificant difference) at 1 year.

In a comprehensive study to characterize dyspareunia, Lowman et al.[23] administered questionnaires to 56 of the sexually active patients who had received a full Prolift mesh surgery. Twenty of the 41 women who responded declared themselves as pain free. Of the 21 patients who reported dyspareunia, 38% (8/21) described their pain as mild, 38% (8/21) as moderate, and 24% (5/21) as severe. These women were not examined to further elucidate the etiology of their pain and their baseline pain is not known. In cohort studies involving mesh repairs, the range of postoperative pain that is not dyspareunia ranges from 0[35] to 20%.[36] Wetta et al.[36] defined pain as any tenderness in the vagina on palpation during examination. They identified 10/50 women with tenderness of which one had a vaginal stricture. It is not known whether the identified pain had an impact on the woman's quality of life. An RTC measuring preoperative and postoperative pelvic pain reported improvement in 15 of 16 women who were treated with mesh for anterior wall prolapse repair compared to 4 of 8 women with native tissue repair.[30] Withagen et al.[18] reported 25% of preoperative women rated their pain as moderately bothered or more. This is compared to 13% total postoperative pain including 5% de novo pain.[18] In a retrospective evaluation of outcomes following different compartment surgery, vaginal pain and bladder pain was seen more commonly in anterior mesh repairs (8% each); and buttock and thigh pain was more common in total vaginal mesh repairs (5% and 2%, respectively).[1] Posterior mesh repairs had the least postoperative pain.

From these studies, it can be generalized that dyspareunia and pelvic pain is often improved following surgery. Mesh use does not appear to affect the total or de novo rates of pain when compared to native tissue repair. This being said, the rate of new onset pain (either pelvic or dyspareunia) appears to be around 5%. This is similar to persistent pain at 1 year following caesarean sections (7%).[21] The overall rate of pain following POP surgery with mesh is less than 20% and closer to

10%. This is similar to persistent pain seen after groin hernia surgery which is reported at a rate of 11% (range 0% to 43%).[28] The identified risk factor for postoperative pain is preoperative pain. Therefore, rates of pain following POP surgery with mesh are similar to other similar surgical procedures.

Role of Mesh in Pain

Usually pain following POP surgery with mesh is attributed to the mesh despite lack of evidence to support this. However, there are studies that have shown how mesh could contribute to unfavorable outcomes. Banding or folding of mesh can cause friction with intercourse with subsequent pain. The vaginal wall may become less pliable as collagen ingrowth occurs. The mesh can retract due to this collagen deposition or due to property changes of the mesh.[32] Vaginal contractures and shortening after mesh placement has been reported. Blandon et al.[3] reported that 48% of patients referred for pain after a vaginal mesh kit had a reduction in vaginal caliber (either a decrease in girth or length). In a retrospective study involving 684 patients, contractures were reported in 3.4% of women having received a total mesh procedure, 5% with posterior mesh only, and 17.6% with anterior mesh.[5] Rogowski et al.[29] showed that women with vaginal pain had larger mesh retraction than those without (35% vs. 10% $p < 0.05$). There was an association between the degree of retraction and the level of pain.[29] If a woman has any restrictions in the pelvic floor musculature prior to surgery and the mesh then contracts, further tension on the musculature can increase presurgery symptoms. The anterior mesh kits pass trocars in the obturator foramen perforating the gracilis and the adductor brevis muscles while the posterior arms perforate the adductor magnus. This can result in ongoing groin pain. Mesh exposures are often associated with pain but can be asymptomatic. This occurs when the mesh is extruded or eroded in the vagina. If this occurs, friction can result in pain and bleeding. Although the mesh can also be extruded in the bladder, urethra, or bowel, this is much less common. These studies support the role of vaginal mesh in producing subsequent pain. The number of women affected in this fashion is not well established. It is also not known which women will be more vulnerable to mesh retraction.

The mesh kits place arms through the sacrospinous ligament for vault fixation. This runs very close to the pudendal nerve and inferior rectal nerve. Studying female cadavers, Castellanos et al.[6] demonstrated the shortest average distance of the trocar of the Prolift Posterior Pelvic Floor Repair System to the pudendal and inferior rectal nerves to be 16.8 mm and 9.7 mm, respectively. The anterior arm of the trocars passes a mean distance from the anterior obturator vessels of 21.2 (SD 1.6) mm on the right side and 20.4 (SD 1.5) mm on the left.[33] The posterior needle passes at a distance to the posterior division of the obturator vessels of 1.8 (SD 1.0) mm on the right side and 1.1 (SD 0.9) mm on the left.[33] As there are anatomical variations and the surgeries are done by palpation and not direct visualization, it is quite easy to imagine that injury would be inevitable. There are no large studies that have reported the rate of nerve or vascular injuries with POP mesh surgery.

Despite nonconfirmatory evidence that mesh causes more pain than native tissue repair, there are compelling studies describing how the mesh can lead to pain. Which women may be at more risk of these complications is unknown. Surgeon experience has been linked to mesh exposures but not to pain.[37]

MANAGEMENT OF PAIN FOLLOWING SURGERY

The literature on management of mesh complications is scarce and limited to retrospective studies.[2] Gyang et al.[16] proposed a stepwise approach beginning with multimodal medical and physical therapy. This approach is the most prudent and likely to lead to more successful outcomes. However, the success of this multimodal approach is not well established. Only after failure to relieve symptoms should release of tension of the mesh be undertaken. This would then be followed by full mesh excision. The rate of mesh excision, full or partial, is not known. However, it can lead to significant morbidity.

In the largest study looking at all mesh excisions for pain, the overall improvement following surgery was 73% (169/233), with 8% (19/233) worsening of pain and 19% (45/233) reporting no change.[8] The presence of chronic pelvic pain prior to the initial surgery was a risk for not improving following mesh excision (OR 0.22, CI 0.12–0.66).[8] Despite different surgical approaches, different initial mesh procedures, and the subjective nature of the pain evaluation, it is important to note that 27% of women did not improve following surgery. Higher failure rates have been reported in smaller cohort studies.[7,19,34]

There are many questions about pain management following surgery that has not been characterized. There does appear to be a cohort of women who will continue to have pain following mesh implantation and explantation. If we use a liberal 20% rate of postoperative pain overall and a 30% failure rate of management of that pain, this leaves 6% of all women operated on who will have pain despite management attempts.

CONCLUSIONS

In 2014, the Medicines and Healthcare products Regulatory Agency (MHRA) in the United Kingdom released its report on adverse events.[26] Monitoring of adverse events depends on voluntary reporting in the United Kingdom by health professionals and the public and mandatory reporting by manufacturers. Pain was reported as 14.6% by health professionals, 28.3% by the public, and 24% by manufactures. Sexual difficulties were reported as 11.2% by health professionals, 15% by the public, and 0% by manufacturers. These reporting variances highlight how stakeholder groups report adverse events differently. Similar shifts were seen in the United States, where a five-fold increase in adverse events reporting was seen on the Manufacturer and User Device Experience (Maude) database following the 2008 FDA statement.[14] In 2016, The FDA reclassified urogynecologic devices from class II to class III, 8 years after its initial statement. This requires manufactures to provide premarketing studies prior to approval.[12]

Over 15 years have elapsed since the first vaginal meshes were introduced in the market. There still remains many unanswered questions and controversy. Could there be any lessons learned from the rise and fall of vaginal meshes? The first is that the introduction of new devices needs to be carefully evaluated prior to general use. This includes not only anatomical success rates and quality of life outcomes, but also complication rates. These can only be addressed by evaluating the pre- and postsurgical changes. Thus, preoperative evaluation needs to be better characterized. Success needs to be balanced with complication rates. Although it is unclear if the complication rates of POP surgery with mesh are higher than that with native tissue repair, there is reason to believe that the mesh itself may contribute to postoperative pain. Even if the complication rates are considered low, the ability to manage postoperative pain effectively is imperative.

REFERENCES

1. Balchandra P, Marsh F, Landon C. Perioperative outcomes and prospective patient reported outcome measures for transvaginal mesh surgery. *Arch Gynecol Obstet.* 2015;292(4):875–882.
2. Barski D, Deng DY. Management of mesh complications after SUI and POP repair: review and analysis of the current literature. *Biomed Res Int.* 2015;2015:831285.
3. Blandon RE, Gebhart JB, Trabuco EC, Klingele CJ. Complications from vaginally placed mesh in pelvic reconstructive surgery. *Int Urogynecol J Pelvic Floor Dysfunct.* 2009;20(5):523–531.
4. Brandsborg B, Nikolajsen L, Hansen CT, Kehlet H, Jensen TS. Risk factors for chronic pain after hysterectomy: a nationwide questionnaire and database study. *Anesthesiology.* 2007;106(5):1003–1012.
5. Caquant F, Collinet P, Debodinance P, et al. Safety of Trans Vaginal Mesh procedure: retrospective study of 684 patients. *J Obstet Gynaecol Res.* 2008;34(4):449–456.
6. Castellanos ME, Yi J, Atashroo D, Desai N, Hibner M. Pudendal neuralgia after posterior vaginal wall repair with mesh kits: an anatomical study and case series. *J Minim Invasive Gynecol.* 2012;19(6):S72–S73.
7. Crosby EC, Abernethy M, Berger MB, DeLancey JO, Fenner DE, Morgan DM. Symptom resolution after operative management of complications from transvaginal mesh. *Obstet Gynecol.* 2014;123(1):134–139.
8. Danford JM, Osborn DJ, Reynolds WS, Biller DH, Dmochowski RR. Postoperative pain outcomes after transvaginal mesh revision. *Int Urogynecol J.* 2015;26(1):65–69.
9. De Tayrac R, Cornille A, Eglin G, et al. Comparison between trans-obturator trans-vaginal mesh and traditional anterior colporrhaphy in the treatment of anterior vaginal wall prolapse: results of a French RCT. *Int Urogynecol J.* 2013;24:1651–1661.

10. Dwyer PL, O'Reilly BA. Transvaginal repair of anterior and posterior compartment prolapse with Atrium polypropylene mesh. *BJOG*. 2004;111(8):831–836.
11. EU Hernia Trialists Collaboration. Repair of groin hernia with synthetic mesh: meta-analysis of randomized controlled trials. *Ann Surg*. 2002;235(3):322–332.
12. Food and Drug Administration. FDA News Release: FDA strengthens requirements for surgical mesh for the transvaginal repair of pelvic organ prolapse to address safety risks. Silver Spring (MD):FDA;2016. Available from https://www.fda.gov/newsevents/newsroom/pressannouncements/ucm479732.htm
13. Food and Drug Administration. FDA public health notification: serious complications associated with transvaginal placement of surgical mesh in repair of pelvic organ prolapse and stress urinary incontinence. Silver Spring (MD): FDA; 2008. Available from http://www.fda.gov/MedicalDevices/Safety/AlertsandNotices/PublicHealthNotifications/ucm061976.htm
14. Food and Drug Administration. FDA safety communication: UPDATE on serious complications associated with transvaginal placement of surgical mesh for pelvic organ prolapse. Silver Spring (MD): FDA; 2011. Available from https://www.fda.gov/downloads/medicaldevices/safety/alertsandnotices/ucm262760.pdf
15. Fränneby U, Sandblom G, Nordin P, Nyrén O, Gunnarsson U. Risk factors for long-term pain after hernia surgery. *Ann Surg*. 2006;244(2):212–219.
16. Gyang AN, Feranec JB, Patel RC, Lamvu GM. Managing chronic pelvic pain following reconstructive pelvic surgery with transvaginal mesh. *Int Urogynecol J*. 2014;25(3):313–318.
17. Handa VL, Garrett E, Hendrix S, Gold E, Robbins J. Progression and remission of pelvic organ prolapse: a longitudinal study of menopausal women. *Am J Obstet Gynecol*. 2004;190(1):27–32.
18. Hendrix SL, Clark A, Nygaard I, Aragaki A, Barnabei V, McTiernan A. Pelvic organ prolapse in the Women's Health Initiative: gravity and gravidity. *Am J Obstet Gynecol*. 2002;186(6):1160–1166.
19. Hokenstad ED, El-Nashar SA, Blandon RE, et al. Health-related quality of life and outcomes after surgical treatment of complications from vaginally placed mesh. *Female Pelvic Med Reconstr Surg*. 2015;21(3):176–180.
20. Jelovsek JE, Barber MD. Women seeking treatment for advanced pelvic organ prolapse have decreased body image and quality of life. *Am J Obstet Gynecol*. 2006;194(5):1455–1461.
21. Jin J, Peng L, Chen Q, et al. Prevalence and risk factors for chronic pain following cesarean section: a prospective study. *BMC Anesthesiol*. 2016;16(1):99.
22. Khandwala S, Jayachandran C. Transvaginal mesh surgery for pelvic organ prolapse—Prolift+ M: a prospective clinical trial. *Int Urogynecol J*. 2011;22(11):1405–1411.

23. Lowman JK, Jones LA, Woodman PJ, Hale DS. Does the Prolift system cause dyspareunia?. *Am J Obstet Gynecol.* 2008;199(6):707.e1–e6.

24. Maher C, Feiner B, Baessler K, Christmann-Schmid C, Haya N, Brown J. Surgery for women with anterior compartment prolapse. *Cochrane Database Syst Rev.* 201611: CD004014.

25. Maher C, Feiner B, Baessler K, Christmann-Schmid C, Haya N, Marjoribanks J. Transvaginal mesh or grafts compared with native tissue repair for vaginal prolapse. *Cochrane Database Syst Rev.* 2016;2:CD012079.

26. Medicines and Healthcare products Regulatory Agency. A summary of the evidence on the benefits and risks of vaginal mesh implants. MRHA:2014. Available from https://www.gov.uk/government/uploads/system/uploads/attachment_data/file/402162/Summary_of_the_evidence_on_the_benefits_and_risks_of_vaginal_mesh_implants.pdf

27. Milani AL, Hinoul P, Gauld JM, Sikirica V, van Drie D, Cosson M; Prolift+M Investigators. Trocar-guided mesh repair of vaginal prolapse using partially absorbable mesh: 1 year outcomes. *Am J Obstet Gynecol.* 2011;204(1):74.e1–e8.

28. Nienhuijs S, Staal E, Strobbe L, Rosman C, Groenewoud H, Bleichrodt R. Chronic pain after mesh repair of inguinal hernia: a systematic review. *Am J Surg.* 2007;194(3):394–400.

29. Rogowski A, Bienkowski P, Tosiak A, Jerzak M, Mierzejewski P, Baranowski W. Mesh retraction correlates with vaginal pain and overactive bladder symptoms after anterior vaginal mesh repair. *Int Urogynecol J.* 2013;24(12):2087–2092.

30. Sivaslioglu AA, Unlubilgin E, Dolen I. A randomized comparison of polypropylene mesh surgery with site-specific surgery in the treatment of cystocoele. *Int Urogynecol J Pelvic Floor Dysfunct.* 2008;19(4):467–471.

31. Smith FJ, Holman CD, Moorin RE, Tsokos N. Lifetime risk of undergoing surgery for pelvic organ prolapse. *Obstet Gynecol.* 2010;116(5):1096–1100.

32. Svabík K, Martan A, Masata J, El-Haddad R, Hubka P, Pavlikova M. Ultrasound appearances after mesh implantation—evidence of mesh contraction or folding? *Int Urogynecol J.* 2011;22(5):529–533.

33. Touboul C, Nizard J, Fauconnier A, Bader G. Perineal approach to vascular anatomy during transobturator cystocele repair. *BJOG.* 2009;116(5):708–712.

34. Unger CA, Abbott S, Evans JM, et al. Outcomes following treatment for pelvic floor mesh complications. *Int Urogynecol J.* 2014;25(6):745–749.

35. Vaiyapuri GR, Han HC, Lee LC, Tseng AL, Wong HF. Retrospective study of transobturator polypropylene mesh kit for the management of pelvic organ prolapse. *Singapore Med J.* 2012;53(10):664–670.

36. Wetta LA, Gerten KA, Wheeler TL, 2nd, Holley RL, Varner RE, Richter HE. Synthetic graft use in vaginal prolapse surgery: objective and subjective outcomes. *Int Urogynecol J Pelvic Floor Dysfunct*. 2009;20(11):1307–1312.
37. Withagen MI, Vierhout ME, Hendriks JC, Kluivers KB, Milani AL. Risk factors for exposure, pain, and dyspareunia after tension-free vaginal mesh procedure. *Obstet Gynecol*. 2011;118(3):629–636.
38. Zondervan K, Barlow DH. Epidemiology of chronic pelvic pain. *Baillieres Best Pract Res Clin Obstet Gynaecol*. 2000;14(3):403–414.

CHAPTER 7

Statins and Pain

John Jarrell

This chapter will focus on the possible mechanisms that result in pain sufficient for subjects to discontinue a medication that can have significant benefits in relation to lipid associated illness. At present there is no consensus as to the actual mechanism of pain from statin medication. The problem is complex. Muscles are affected by many conditions confounding the diagnosis of statin related disease. The metabolism of statins is complicated by variations in transporter systems in liver and muscle tissue as well as interaction with a host of medications that makes a unified theory of pain mechanism possible at present. This summary will provide an overview of the problem. For detailed elaboration of the complex biochemistry of statins, muscle physiology and possible mechanisms of muscle pain, as well as approaches to alternative therapy, the reader is referred to recent and excellent detailed texts.[8,20,25]

STATIN MEDICATION

Statin medications are considered by some to be the most effective approach to prevent and treat cardiovascular disease.[8] It is estimated that approximately 25% of the world's population over the age of 65 years is taking a statin for primary or secondary prevention of this condition.[14] This concept is not shared by all however. The administration of statin medication is based on the cholesterol hypothesis wherein dietary cholesterol is responsible for cardiovascular disease. This has been challenged more recently based on a number of different approaches.[9] Although this chapter is not designed to enter the statin controversy it is important to indicate there are concerns regarding the medication and its benefits. These concerns can be summarized as the following: The association of cholesterol to heart disease does not equal causation, the early statin trials are potentially flawed, mortality rates are more relevant in the determination of effectiveness in the prevention of cardiovascular disease, meta-analysis from the Cochrane database indicates while statins are beneficial in reducing cardiovascular event, there was no change in mortality and finally, the Mediterranean diet is acknowledged as a means toward improved mortality rates without changes in cholesterol.

There is a wide spectrum of clinical consequence from the administration of statins. Most patients appear to be asymptomatic while muscle pain affects a minority in a variety of ways. Due to widespread appreciation of the controversy regarding statins, there is legitimate concern that the pain from stain administration may reflect a true nocebo effect. Muscle pain is generally reported as bilaterally symmetrical in the proximal muscles of the upper and lower extremities. In some there is an asymptomatic release of creatine kinase measurable in the serum while in others the symptoms evolve to myalgia (muscle pain or weakness), myositis (muscle pain or weakness with elevation of creatine kinase), or rarely rhabdomyolysis (muscle pain and weakness with high levels of creatine kinase, myoglobinuria, possible renal failure and death).[16] The rates of muscle pain associated with statins are varied due in part to difficulty in clarity of diagnosis and the fact that early clinical trials were not designed to assess this as an outcome measure.[5] The reported rates of muscle pain range from 7% to 29% and the problem is a common cause of discontinuation of the medication.[18,37] A classification of the phenotypes of statin-induced myotoxicity has been proposed (Table 7-1).[1] In most cases of SIM 0–1 the medication is continued but in more severe forms the drug is discontinued with recovery for most except SIM6 when the symptoms persist.[37]

TABLE 7-1 **Statin-Induced Myotoxicity (SIM) Classification and Prevalence**

Classification	Phenotype	Prevalence
SIM 0	CK elevation <4 × ULN No Myalgia	1.5–26%
SIM 1	CK not elevated Mild myalgia	0.3–33%
SIM 2	CK elevated <4 × ULN Severe myalgia	0.2–20%
SIM 3	CK >10 × ULN <10 × ULN Myopathy	5/100,000
SIM 4	CK >10 × ULN <50 × ULN Severe myopathy	0.11%
SIM 5	CK >10 × ULN Rhabdomyolysis	0.1–8.4/100,000 Patients per year
SIM 6	HMG-CoAR antibodies Autoimmune-mediated necrotizing myositis	2/1,000,000 patients Per year

EARLY RECOGNITION OF AN ASSOCIATION WITH PAIN

An early recording of pain resulting from a statin was in a placebo-controlled trial of mevinolin administration that resulted in significant decreases of cholesterol and while the drug was reported to be well tolerated there was one subject withdrawn because of abdominal pain.[38] Subsequent reports of pain were made in 1990 indicating the administration of a statin could be associated with abdominal pain, cramps, bloating, and flatus in 4% to 6% of cases.[6] In a placebo trial of simvastatin, the active drug was stopped in one patient (abdominal pain, dizziness, headache, and tiredness) and in two patients taking the placebo (elevated creatine phosphokinase, cardiovascular collapse).[24] Another early report of muscular side effects was made by England.[11]

Interestingly, muscle issues also emerged with reports of rhabdomyolysis in association with the administration of lovastatin. The FDA noted 12 case reports of severe myopathy or rhabdomyolysis associated with concomitant use of lovastatin and gemfibrozil in which serum creatine kinase levels were more than 10,000 U/L, with associated myoglobinuria, and acute renal failure. For the first year of marketing of lovastatin, spontaneous reports of myopathy with documentation of creatine kinase level were reviewed for the use of lovastatin, gemfibrozil, and combination therapy. The median creatine kinase level in reports involving concomitant lovastatin and gemfibrozil use was 15,250 U/L, 20 times that in reports with gemfibrozil use alone and 30 times that in reports with lovastatin use alone. Because of the potential for severe myopathy and life-threatening rhabdomyolysis, and given alternative drug combinations for treating hyperlipoproteinemia, the use of lovastatin in combination with gemfibrozil is to be discouraged.[28] The first reports were associated with the coadministration of statin with cyclosporine, gemfibrozil, nicotinic acid, and erythromycin.[2,7,10,13,25,30,36] Among the first reports of rhabdomyolysis the authors speculated that the disorder was due to mitochondrial damage secondary to inadequate synthesis of coenzyme Q and heme A, members of the electron-transport system of the inner mitochondrial membrane.[20] The clinical course was characterized by profound muscle weakness increase in serum creatine kinase and myoglobin. Light- and electron-microscopic studies of skeletal muscle demonstrated a noninflammatory myopathy suggestive of ongoing rhabdomyolysis with vacuolization and focal degeneration of myocytes. Symptoms and the laboratory values resolved after discontinuation of the drug.[20]

BIOCHEMISTRY OF STATINS

Statin-induced pain is often but not always associated with increased levels of the specific drug or metabolites in the serum, indicating the mechanism of pain involves both pharmacokinetic conditions as well as muscle accumulation of the drug.[27] Once absorbed from the intestine, statins are required to enter the liver, undergo transformation to affect their metabolic action and are then eliminated. Statins are absorbed into the hepatocyte by membrane carrier polypeptides. Once inside the hepatocyte, lovastatin and simvastatin are converted to hydroxylated metabolites by the cytochrome P450 and then act to competitively inhibit 3-hydroxy-3-methylglutaryl-coenzyme A reductase (HMG-CoAR). In order to generate muscle injury the statins must enter and accumulate in muscle tissue. Entry is effected through influx transporters balanced by efflux transporters.

MUSCLE PHYSIOLOGY

The energy of muscle action depends on the availability of ATP that is generated in the mitochondria through cellular respiration. Pyruvate formed from glucose and lactate is oxidized in the mitochondria and oxidized to Acetyl CoA that is then incorporated into the tricarboxylic acid cycle reduced to B-nicotinamide adenine dinucleotide (NADH which is then oxidized to generate ATP). ATP is also formed in the muscle by the phosphorylation of ADP as well as from ketone bodies when glucose availability is limited. In the mitochondrion, reactive oxygen species play a role in cellular respiration. Active exercise increases the production of peroxide that results in a stimulation in production of superoxide dismutase, catalase, and glutathione peroxidase that decrease the reactive oxidative species.

Muscles and Pain

In muscle biopsies of patients with SIM there is mitochondrial dysfunction, reduced production of ATP, enhanced production of reactive oxygen species, and apoptosis with disordered calcium metabolism. Statins can be shown to alter the integrity of the sarcoplasma and the mitochondria.[21] The statin action can be indirect or direct. Indirectly the inhibition of HMG-CoAR is associated with several possible explanations for the emergence of SIM: reduction in mevalonate, reduction in ubiquinone, induction of apoptosis, and an increase in proteolysis.[4,12,15,26,34]

Direct effects of statins on the myocyte include depression of the mitochondrial respiratory chain, dysregulation of calcium metabolism, and muscle remodeling.[17,19,35]

Muscle nociception is transmitted to the spinal cord though unmyelinated C fibers and myelinated A Delta fibers.[21] The nociceptors are responsive to ATP, bradykinin, serotonin, substance P, histamine, prostaglandin E2, and capsaicin. The tissues are also responsive to calcium and an acidic environment Graven. Lactate also stimulates chemosensitive afferent fibers.[33] Muscle pain during exercise is due to the accumulation of lactate.[31] The administration of protons, lactate, and ATP provokes fatigue and pain in volunteers.[29,40] Increased lactate and ADP and diminished calcium have been associated with muscle fatigue and pain.[39]

TREATMENT

The treatment approaches to statin-induced pain are directed to discontinuing the drug on a temporary basis and reintroducing the drug through a variety of treatment options. Although muscle pain is the most common adverse effect from statin usage, in many cases it has been shown the symptoms are from other forms of musculoskeletal disorders. Randomized trials have shown there are similar rates of muscle pain complaints among those on statins and those receiving a placebo.[32] It is therefore important to determine if the symptom is truly associated with a statin medication through assessment of creatine kinase levels and careful readministration approaches. The common complaint associated with SAMS (statin associated myopathy) is a dull aching in the proximal muscles of the leg and arm. With this or a similar presentation the clinician should undertake a review of the clinical indication if this has not been a part of the original decision to implement statin therapy. Efforts should be made to either determine if the complaints of pain are either not due to the statin or to identify if true intolerance exists. Recommended approaches have included candid patient counseling, shared decision making, eliminating contributing factors, reduced dosage, alternate statin medication, gradual reintroduction of the drug, and intermittent dosing.[3] This is done using different approaches to reintroduction of the drug following a 2-week washout period and implementing intermittent dosing.[3] If intolerance is identified, important coexistent illness should be explored such as hypothyroidism and some muscle abnormalities such as polymyalgia rheumatic. Clinical factors associated with statin intolerance are presented in Table 7-2. A greater number of factors indicate a greater risk of myopathy. High concentrations of statin in the blood are associated with greater rates of adverse outcomes. Polypharmacy is also a possible risk for administration of drugs that act to increase statin concentrations: medication(s) that inhibit cytochrome P450 (CYP450) isoenzymes, organic anion transport protein 1B1 (OATP1B1), or P-glycoprotein 1 (P-gp) have been associated with increased risk of new or worsening muscle pain.[37]

TABLE 7-2 Clinical Risk Factors of Statin-Induced Myopathy[3,22,37]

Older patients >75 years
Female
Asian ethnicity
Frailty
Pre-existing musculoskeletal disorders
Chronic pain
Diabetes mellitus
Chronic renal or hepatic disease
Hypothyroidism
Human immunodeficiency disease
Vitamin D deficiency
Severe trauma
Family history of myalgia
Physical exertion
Pharmacologic agents increasing statin concentration
Amiodarone
Azole antifungal agents
Cyclosporine
Gemfibrozil
Diltiazem
Verapamil
Erythromycin clarithromycin
Protease inhibitors
Grapefruit in large quantities
Related history
History of creatine kinase elevation, especially 10× the upper limit of the normal range
History of pre-existing/unexplained muscle/joint/tendon pain
Inflammatory or inherited metabolic, neuromuscular/muscle defects (e.g., McArdle disease, carnitine palmitoyltransferase II deficiency, myoadenylate deaminase deficiency, and malignant hyperthermia)
Previous statin-induced myotoxicity
History of myopathy while receiving another lipid-lowering therapy
Genetics
Genetic polymorphisms encoding cytochrome P450 isoenzymes or drug transporters
Other risk factors
High level of physical activity
Dietary effects (excessive grapefruit or cranberry juice)
Excess alcohol
Drug abuse (cocaine, amphetamines, heroin)

Despite this approach there is considerable information suggesting that muscle pain can continue well after the discontinuation of the drug. While this may be due to nocebo concerns or alternative musculoskeletal disorders, it remains a problem to determine the mechanism of pain more fully. Whenever there is doubt regarding the diagnosis, muscle biopsy may be of help as shown in Figure 7-1.[23]

Modification of the diet is recommended to include a low saturated fat diet and avoidance of trans fats, consumption of viscous fiber (mainly psyllium, 10 g daily) and foods with added plant sterols or stanols (2 g daily) has also been shown to reduce LDL-C by 7% and 10%, respectively.[37]

In addition to these general principles, a flow chart of approaches depending on the severity of the condition has been developed by the European Atherosclerosis Society (Table 7-3).

TABLE 7-3 **Management of the Patient with SAMS and Statin Administration**

Muscle pain, creatine kinase <4× Normal

- Low risk –
  - consider changing lifestyle activities in lieu of statin
- High risk –
  - rechallenge or change to an alternative statin

Muscle pain, creatine kinase >4× Normal

- Low risk –
  - stop statin and reassess need
  - Lower dose of alternative statin
- High risk
  - Statin can be continued but monitor CK values
  - If greater than 10 × ULN they should be discontinued and a lower dose of alternate statin used

Muscle pain CK values >10 × ULN

- Discontinue statin
- Consider alternative drug a lower dose following CK

Adapted from Stroes ES, Thompson PD, Corsini A, et al.; European Atherosclerosis Society Consensus Panel. Statin-associated muscle symptoms: impact on statin therapy-European Atherosclerosis Society Consensus Panel Statement on Assessment, Aetiology and Management. *Eur Heart J.* 2015;36(17):1012–1022.

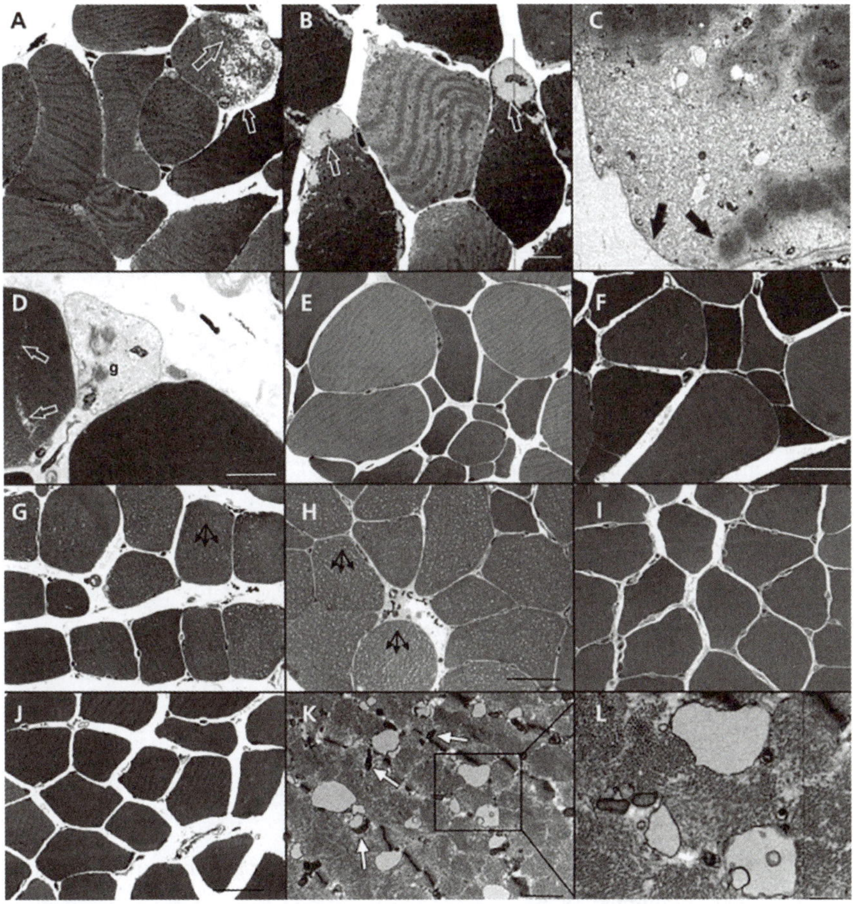

FIGURE 7-1 Skeletal muscle injury in patients with statin-associated myopathy. Light micrographs **(A, B, D, E, F)** and an electron micrograph **(C)** of transverse sections through the vastus lateralis muscle of patients with myopathy and current **(B, D, E, F)** or previous **(A, C)** statin use. Subsarcolemmal detachment of myofibrils is indicated by *arrows* in **(A)**, **(B)**, and **(C)**. In **(D)**, a ghost cell *(g)* is seen next to a developing split-fiber (*arrows*). **(G, H):** Light micrographs of semi-thin, transverse sections through the vastus lateralis muscle of myopathic patients currently **(G)** or formerly taking statins **(H)**. Vacuolization is seen in most of the fibers (*arrows*). **(I, J):** The muscles fibers from control patients show no vacuolization. **(K, L):** Electron micrographs of a transverse section through the vastus lateralis muscle from a patient with myopathy who formerly used statins; intracellular vacuoles are present. The boxed area in **(K)** is enlarged in **(L)**. The T-tubules are grossly vacuolated, but the adjacent mitochondria (m) have a normal appearance. Bars: A, B = 10 μm; C = 0.2 μm; D = 3 μm; E, F = 50 μm; G, I, J = 50 μm, H = 30 μm, K = 1 μm; L = 0.5 μm. (From Mohaupt MG, Karas RH, Babiychuk EB, et al. Association between statin-associated myopathy and skeletal muscle damage. *CMAJ*. 2009;181(1–2):E11–E18.).

CONCLUSION

The problem of statin-related pain remains an open challenge for the clinician to determine its presence, severity, and management approaches that establish the best possible safety. There remains a challenge for those involved in pain physiology to determine if there is a universal theory for the onset and continuation of statins that can occur even following discontinuation of the drug.

REFERENCES

1. Alfirevic A, Neely D, Armitage J, et al. Phenotype standardization for statin-induced myotoxicity. *Clin Pharmacol Ther*. 2014;96(4):470–476.
2. Ayanian JZ, Fuchs CS, Stone RM. Lovastatin and rhabdomyolysis. *Ann Intern Med*. 1988;109(8):682–683.
3. Backes JM, Ruisinger JF, Gibson CA, Moriarty PM. Statin-associated muscle symptoms—Managing the highly intolerant. *J Clin Lipidol*. 2017;11(1):24–33.
4. Banach M, Mikhailidis DP; Lipid and Blood Pressure Meta-analysis Collaboration (LBPMC) Group. In reply–Coenzyme Q10 and statin-induced myopathy. *Mayo Clin Proc*. 2015;90(3):420–421.
5. Bays H. Statin safety: an overview and assessment of the data - 2005. *Am J Cardiol*. 2006;97(8A):6c–26c.
6. Bilheimer DW. Long-term clinical tolerance of lovastatin and simvastatin. *Cardiology*. 1990;77 (Suppl 4):58–65.
7. Blaison G, Weber JC, Sachs D, et al. [Rhabdomyolysis caused by simvastatin a patient following heart transplantation and cyclosporine therapy]. *Rev Med Interne*. 1992;13(1):61–63.
8. Du Souich P, Roederer G, Dufour R. Myotoxicity of statins: mechanism of action. *Pharmacol Ther*. 2017;175:1–16.
9. DuBroff R, de Lorgeril M. Cholesterol confusion and statin controversy. *World J Cardiol*. 2015;7(7):404–409.
10. East C, Alivizatos PA, Grundy SM, Jones PH, Farmer JA. Rhabdomyolysis in patients receiving lovastatin after cardiac transplantation. *N Engl J Med*. 1988;318(1):47–48.
11. England JD, Viles A, Walsh JC, Stewart PM. Muscle side effects associated with simvastatin therapy. *Med J Aust*. 1990;153(9):562–563.

12. Gee RH, Spinks JN, Malia JM, Johnston JD, Plant NJ, Plant KE. Inhibition of prenyltransferase activity by statins in both liver and muscle cell lines is not causative of cytotoxicity. *Toxicology.* 2015;329:40–48.
13. Goldman JA, Fishman AB, Lee JE, Johnson RJ. The role of cholesterol-lowering agents in drug-induced rhabdomyolysis and polymyositis. *Arthritis Rheum.* 1989;32(3):358359.
14. Gu Q, Paulose-Ram R, Burt VL, Kit BK. Prescription cholesterol-lowering medication use in adults aged 40 and over: United States, 2003–2012. *NCHS Data Brief.* 2014; 177:1–8.
15. Johnson TE, Zhang X, Bleicher KB, et al. Statins induce apoptosis in rat and human myotube cultures by inhibiting protein geranylgeranylation but not ubiquinone. *Toxicol Appl Pharmacol.* 2004;200(3):237–250.
16. Joy TR, Hegele RA. Narrative review: statin-related myopathy. *Ann Intern Med.* 2009;150(12):858–868.
17. Kaufmann P, Torok M, Zahno A, Waldhauser KM, Brecht K, Krahenbuhl S. Toxicity of statins on rate skeletal muscle mitochondria. *Cell Mol Life Sci.* 2006;63(19–20): 2415–2425.
18. Khan A, Maki KC, Ito MK. Ito MK. Statin associated muscle symptoms: characteristics of patients and recommendations by providers. *J Clin Lipidol.* 2015;9(3):460.
19. Kwak HB, Thalacker-Mercer A, Anderson EJ, et al. Simvastatin impairs ADP-stimulated respiration and increases mitochondrial oxidative stress in primary human skeletal myotubes. *Free Radic Biol Med.* 2012;52(1):198–207.
20. Manoukian AA, Bhagavan NV, Hayashi T, Nestor TA, Rios C, Scottolini AG. Rhabdomyolysis secondary to lovastatin therapy. *Clin Chem.* 1990;36(12):2145–2147.
21. Millan J, Pedro-Botet J, Climent E, Millan J, Rius J. [Statin associated myopathy in clinical practice. Results of DAMA study]. *Clin Investig Arterioscler.* 2017;29(1): 7–12.
22. Mobhammer D, Schaeffler E, Scwab M, Morike K. Mechanisms and assessment of statin-related muscular adverse effects. *Br J Clin Pharmacol.* 2014;78(3):454–466.
23. Mohaupt MG, Karas RH, Babiychuk EB, et al. Association between statin-associated myopathy and skeletal muscle damage. *CMAJ.* 2009;181(1–2):E11–E18.
24. Morgan T, Anderson A, McDonald P, Hopper J, Macaskill G. Simvastatin in the treatment of hypercholesterolaemia in patients with essential hypertension. *J Hypertens Suppl.* 1990;8(1):S25–S30.
25. Norman DJ, Illingworth DR, Munson J, Hosenpud J. Myolysis and acute renal failure in a heart transplant recipient receiving lovastatin. *N Engl J Med.* 1988;318(1): 46–47.

26. Osaki Y, Nakagawa Y, Miyahara S, et al. Skeletal muscle-specific HMG-CoA reductase knockout mice exhibit rhabdomyolysis: A model for statin-induced myopathy. *Biochem Biophys Res Commun.* 2015;466(3):536–540.

27. Philips PS, Haas RH, Bannykh S, et al.; Scripps Mercy Clinical Research Center. Statin-induced myopathy with normal creatine kinase l levels. *Ann Intern Med.* 2002;137(7):581–585.

28. Pierce LR, Wysowski DK, Gross TP. Myopathy and rhabdomyolysis associated with lovastatin-gemfibrozil combination therapy. *JAMA.* 1990;264(1):71–75.

29. Pollak KA, Swenson JD, Vanhaitsma TA, et al. Exogenously applied muscle metabolites synergistically evoke sensations of muscle fatigue and pain in human subjects. *Exp Phys.* 2014;99:368–380.

30. Reaven P, Witztum JL. Lovastatin, nicotinic acid, and rhabdomyolysis. *Ann Intern Med.* 1988;109(7):597–598.

31. Rosendal L, Larsson B, Kristiansen J, et al. Increase in muscle nociceptive substances and anaerobic metabolism in patients with trapezius myalgia: microdialysis in rest and during exercise. *Pain.* 2004;112(3):324–334.

32. Rosenson RS, Baker S, Banach M, et al. Optimizing cholesterol treatment in patients with muscle complaints. *J Am Coll Cardiol.* 2017;70(10):1290–1301.

33. Rotto DM, Kaufman MP. Effect of metabolic products of muscular contraction on discharge of group III and group IV afferents. *J Appl Physiol (1985).* 1988;64(6):2306–2313.

34. Sakamoto K, Kimura J. Mechanism of statin-induced rhabdomyolysis. *J Pharmacol Sci.* 2013;123(4):289–294.

35. Sirvent P, Mercier J, Vassort G, Lacampagne A. Simvastatin triggers mitochondria-induced Ca2+ signaling alteration in skeletal muscle. *BBRC.* 2005;329(3):1067–1075.

36. Spach DH, Bauwens JE, Clark CD, Burke WG. Rhabdomyolysis associated with lovastatin and erythromycin use. *West J Med.* 1991;154(2):213–215.

37. Stroes ES, Thompson PD, Corsini A, et al.; European Atherosclerosis Society Consensus Panel. Statin-associated muscle symptoms: impact on statin therapy-European Atherosclerosis Society Consensus Panel Statement on Assessment, Aetiology and Management. *Eur Heart J.* 2015;36(17):1012–1022.

38. Tobert JA, Bell GD, Birtwell J, et al. Cholesterol-lowering effect of mevinolin, an inhibitor of 3-hydroxy-3-methylglutaryl-coenzyme a reductase, in healthy volunteers. *J Clin Invest.* 1982;69(4):913–919.

39. Vandenbloom R. The myofibrillar complex and fatigue: a review. *Can J Appl Physiol.* 2004;29:330–356.

40. Wang K, Luo Y, Asaki T, et al. Acid-induced experimental muscle pain and hyperalgesia with single and repeated infusion in human forearm. *Scand J Pain.* 2017;17:260–266.

INDEX